# Why You Can't Have Your Cake & Eat It Too.

## *Food-Borne Illness*

## By Nadine Campbell, R. N.

**Published By**
*NutriStrat Press™*
*Tempe, Arizona*

Copyright 2005 © Nadine Campbell, R. N. NutriStrat Press



ISBN #0-9771590-1-9

**NutriStrat Press**
**Tempe, Arizona**
WWW.nutritionalstrategist.com
strategicqueendw@aol.com

**Printed In The United States Of America**

## Dedication

To all those who have tried and failed at this thing we call a diet. To all those who have started and stopped because they lost hope before they lost weight. To all the flip-flops, loafers, and slippers who stop before they can start making a "diet" work.

To all the quick fixes, and the procrastinators; which are the two sides of the same coin. To the magic pill, the super food, and green tea extract which have not enriched your life as much as they have enriched the cash drawers of the stores.

We are tossed this way and that with each new nutritional infomercial or trend. Clever marketing has blunted the directional signal that usually guides our appetites. The constant bombardment of media-based advertising is much like the old propaganda machines named Tokyo Rose and Hanoi Jane. We cannot discern good information from the hard sell.

Our nutritional belief systems have bound us in many ways. Now we are unhealthy and over-fat, or we are unhealthy and underweight. False belief systems act like strings attached to each one of us. We have become puppets jerking to whatever whim the market chooses. We believed there was something lacking in us when the reality was we were enough.

This book is dedicated to changing a global perception about nutrition for the human body. We cannot afford to weight. We cannot afford to wait. It is time to change the energy.

Blessings, Nadine Campbell

To

# Gretel

12-20-1990 to 6-28-2005

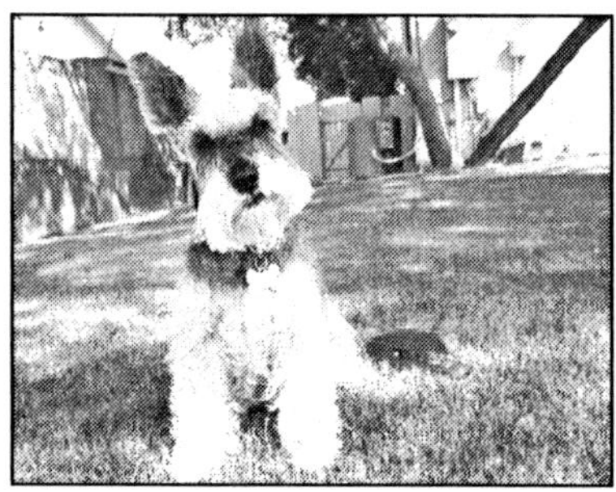

## My little angel…

# Introduction

There are three rules of the universe. One is: You have to look before you leap. Two: You cannot have your cake and eat it too. Three: There is no substitute for hard work.

There are many fabrications abroad, but these basic concepts are applicable to all levels of life. In case you haven't noticed, societies all over the planet are suffering from either too much food or not enough. The effects of these forms of malnutrition are disease, disability, and death. We are on a track to extinction simply because our nutrition and hydration states are so poor.

The primary reason we eat so poorly is the result of the extreme programming civilization has been exposed to for the last fifty years. The perceptions we have generated are for the most part false, because the premises of the programmers are flawed. Our culture is like a giant computer with a Trojan horse virus corrupting all its intelligence when it comes to nutrition.

For all the wonderful technology created to improve life as we know it, humanity will extinguish itself because of its behavior with food.

We need to change our perceptions about protein and water. These two important elements have become stigmatized as undesirables. Human nutrition is dependent on protein, fat, carbohydrates, and water. We need it all, but just not the way the food "pyramids" would have us believe. The significance of the food pyramid on the culture of eating has been a complete disaster.

# Why You Can't Have Your Cake & Eat It, Too: Food Borne Illness

Not only is the food pyramid difficult to understand, but also it represents the special interests of the food industries, reaching their long arm into our wallets. This wallet-surgery extends to our health, health care, and the cost of doing business. With 60% of the work force chronically ill, the cost to commerce and the family is extraordinary. The most dangerous pathogen to public health is food, in the way it is generally misunderstood.

The ideas presented here are to challenge the sacred cows of nutrition. These sacred cows are low-fat mentality, calorie counting, portion control, and exercise as a way to get healthy and lose weight. The food pyramid is the biggest sacred cow of all. In order to change the obesity/malnutrition epidemic we have to be willing to sacrifice these sacred cows, get rid of them and never create any new ones.

# Table of Contents

# Why You Can't Have Your Cake & Eat It, Too: Food Borne Illness

# Preface

This textbook is compiled from the experience I have accumulated over the course of my journey through the mysteries of eating. I managed to gain and lose the same ten pounds many times over. Twice I gained and lost 30 pounds. I worked as an aerobic dance instructor for five years, and still had trouble managing my weight... I was a loyal member of a couple of weight-loss enterprises, with the same results. This is humbling and hard work!

I began to see that one's resistances to life and change run parallel to resistances taking place in the physical body. I began to see a correlation between stubbornness and physical sickness. Moreover, intellectual inflexibility as a strong oppositional force appeared to be a part of the entire dynamic. Many forms of emotional resistance manifest in physical illness. It is possible to express resistance to change as discomfort and disease. On some occasions the manner in which these resistances are "languaged" to the person may inspire true change, even acceptance. Our insides show up on our outsides. Our internal resistances, be they physical, emotional or spiritual, are reflected in our state of health. Well-being is a mirror of our health on all levels.

Generating a state of physical health is an invaluable tool while navigating a course through life. Even if depression, economic challenges, or illness become part of the individual's dynamic, being in top physical condition has relevance to the effort of becoming a bold participant in those struggles.

## Why You Can't Have Your Cake & Eat It, Too

Our country is becoming more physically disabled. Why is this? We are enjoying more technology, more information, and more abundance. It would seem that humanity is perpetually destined to shoot itself in the foot. The belief systems we hold about nutrition are not working. Many of these ideas contain no scientific truth whatsoever, yet we fiercely resist giving them up. We might even be horrified that someone would attack the food pyramid, not realizing that this is just one example of an erroneous belief system.

These erroneous belief systems also represent economic and political interests. Many commercial institutions are heavily invested in government endorsements which, in turn, are veiled as pseudo-science. These belief systems are based on economics, with human physiology as the last consideration. Even proving these belief systems false results in very little change in public health policy. This is public policy resistance. Those who dare challenge the status quo of these nutritional belief systems can endure dire consequences. The laws that protect the food industry from criticism leave the FDA and the USDA helpless against the commercial enterprises they are supposed to be overseeing. This is the bottom line.

The statistics on health-related consequences of obesity are indicative of a slow, steady decline in the health of our country. We think of people starving in Third World countries, but fail to acknowledge the malnutrition on our shores. The paradox of the over-fed and the under-fed represent the malnutrition we like to forget. The chance of becoming overweight and sick is over 60% for all populations. This is a form of malnutrition. Yet we fail to see it and sound the alarm.

## Why You Can't Have Your Cake & Eat It, Too

This problem is affecting youngsters, who are acquiring the diseases of maturity at a dizzying pace.

This is a public health crisis. It is an epidemic. It is a pandemic. We are told over and over the same thing: eat less and exercise more. This is just the beginning of the false belief systems we have about nutrition. There are more. We will explore these false belief systems and begin to understand their purpose. Then slowly, the language of nutritional wisdom will be revealed to you. Your mystery, your "why", will be explained in terms you can understand. The mythologies you have used to help you interpret your current reality are wishful thinking. They are keeping you stuck, sick, and tired.

Your new understanding will give you the education you need to change what may seem like a hopeless situation. You have already tried everything else. What have you got to lose? Let's find out.

Joy on the journey to wellness,

Nadine Campbell, R.N.

# Why You Can't Have Your Cake & Eat It, Too

## Chapter One:
## Waiting/Weighting is Optional

Becoming well, getting healthy, is an ongoing challenge. Various degrees of health-related changes require constant adaptation. Confronting our on-going health issues head-on is best. Our culture has significant tribal-like beliefs governing nutrition and health. These belief systems control the government of healing and regulate the speed at which we are permitted to heal. More importantly, these same belief systems insure the survival of the food and drug monopolies.

Resistance patterns appear internally and externally. Rigid, closely-held belief systems often parallel cellular resistance. Much writing on this topic discusses insulin resistance and ways to diminish it. Involving the entire mind/body/spirit in the effort to obtain a state of health and wellness is very important. An examination of each belief system will be helpful in releasing some of our intellectual, emotional, and spiritual resistance, because our internal dialogue often reflects our deeply-held resistances. It is helpful to address your particular repetitious themes.

Resistance is a form of weight/wait held on the body. Ambiguity, procrastination, justifications, comparisons, judgments, anger, depression, avoidance, and over-indulgences are examples of resistance strategies. As the body manifests real life symptoms, it is interesting to note the parallels in very specific symptoms, often requiring medical intervention. Today's medical interventions address the symptoms. This book will address the causes of insulin resistance and ways to improve it.

# Why You Can't Have Your Cake & Eat It, Too

The techniques presented here are designed to be flexible to meet the needs of each individual. Travel, family celebrations, vegetarianism, and eating out will be addressed. This is a very specific individual process. Family members have differing degrees of tolerances to food values. Tailoring an eating plan just for you is the most important aspect of this effort. Second in importance is doing the nutritional program every day, no matter what the circumstances. This will mean looking up food values, keeping food records, monitoring mood, and documenting blood sugars when indicated. Checking in with your health professional for any status changes is a part of the process. You must realize that this is something at which you will have to work. Education and understanding are not enough.

The impact of circumstances on our life can trigger a form of weight/wait. This is procrastination, the deadliest force in the work of getting healthy. The unexpected tolerances for food values in your diet will demand constant adaptations to your plans. Each time we say, "This I will not give up", we are practicing resistance. Those little hold-outs will add wait/weight to the effort. Insulin resistance, like other resistances, does not just go away. It can become manageable, provided one is willing to monitor one's physical status on a daily basis. You cannot possibly outrun these consequences.

We can improve your health. It is true. This improvement happens at the speed of acceptance. What you resist persists. Want what you have. Want it fully. Choose with integrity. The choices you make really matter and your life may depend on them.

# Why You Can't Have Your Cake & Eat It, Too

Language is very interesting to me. Words that sound the same, but have different meanings always get my attention. I am particularly attached to three words. They are way, weight, and wait. There is a synchronicity in how these words relate to the health mystery of insulin resistance and obesity. It is my observation that when we are overweight, we over-wait. I note how many days and weeks go by with a life put on hold. I see folks isolate, being weighted with their burdens. I see them put all kinds of conditions on the effort they are willing to maintain (wait). Procrastination is right up there, too, as a form of wait. It adds to the weight.

The area of finances is particularly affected by waiting. We speak of being weighted by debt. Often we put off doing something until we have enough money. We may believe that one process is going to be more expensive than another. We will dismiss a good idea prior to investigation simply because it might cost too much. One of the resistances I hear about is not having enough money to afford something perhaps food or medication. However, if one carefully reviewed how one finances his life, he may find new ways of using the money he already has. In other words, there is always enough money for video games or cigarettes, but not enough to buy tuna fish.

Here is the way to weigh. Here is the wait in weight. Interestingly, the words give us some new views. Using weigh, way, and wait interchangeably is a helpful tool we can use to describe how we relate to our procrastination. When life makes sense to us, we usually don't want to change anything. We can move forward and feel comfortable. When life doesn't make sense we tend to put on the brakes. We wait in the why spot. Perhaps we need to move forward, make our own way, but we wait until we have a fully detailed explanation for why things have happened the way they have. We refuse to go into the unknown territory of our life. We weight/wait. If we have used all of our nutritional and exercise mythology to outrun our health-related consequences, our mystery deepens when we get sick or obese. We give up, and we wait. Even if the motor is at idle, it requires fuel. It is wait, weight.

Removing obstacles is a perfect image for weight. Observe your space. Is it chaotic with everything piled around? These piles are little pieces of weight. They are your history, also known as the weight of history. As our history grows, we hold onto it. These accumulations should be called 'stuffology'. "Stuffologists" often try to hide their stuff, and this effort takes a lot of energy. Especially difficult to hide is a food addiction. Should one over-consume or under-consume food, the results of these habits become obvious. Yet, most "stuffologists" will be oblivious to their physical condition. This is called denial.

There are stuffologists who have the pack-rat habit. They cannot give up anything. It takes a lot of mental constructions to support this inability to let go of old stuff. Huge piles of collected stuff slowly become unmovable obstacles which are in the way, just adding to the weight, and the wait. The physical objects are easy to spot for the space they occupy. These are symbolic of the weight and the wait and represent two problems. One problem involves money and the other involves time. Sometimes we have to pay for all of this stuff and paying for it is going to take time. It will also provide lots of distraction, another form of procrastination.

What about this chaos? What are you waiting for? Who are you waiting for? How long will it take? Are we there yet?

# Why You Can't Have Your Cake & Eat It, Too

Being "less than truthful" is a politically correct phrase to describe the habit of omission. Lying in weight. Telling lies is a profound form of self-sabotage. It requires a lot of energy to keep track of the tangled web we weave. The purpose of being less than truthful is to avoid personal responsibility for the choices you make. Remember the old adage: "It is a poor carpenter who blames his tools." Hiding, sneaking, slipping, and sliding gives the illusion of applying a brake to the speed of time. Remember, this is an illusion because there is a tremendous amount of energy exerted to keep things the way they are. What then? Isolation and unavailability are usually employed. Sometimes this is a brake. Sometimes it is an obstacle. It represents a way to control change by holding on to what we need to believe.

Inertia is another form of wait/weight. Think of it as two opposing forces pushing with all their might. We might think we are waiting, but we are using a lot of energy to maintain the status quo. This is another type of justification. Perhaps we will say we just need to maintain for a while. Change is a constant, steady form of energy. It does not wait. Imagine standing on a stepping-stone in the middle of a stream and telling yourself that you are going to stay there until you have solved all of your mysteries. You may wobble back and forth in an effort to keep your balance. After many days of holding your position on that rock in the middle of the stream, exhaustion or a lack of energy begins. Gingerly you might pick out a nearby stone to settle on, but you don't have the power within you to get there. Your energy has been expended on holding your position. You fear getting wet in the cool water of the stream. Inertia is just like that. It takes loads of energy to go nowhere while you maintain a holding pattern. You might as well just get wet, learn to swim, and learn to navigate the belief systems that bind you.

Sometimes we carry around the problems of our families and friends, like weight on our back, our shoulders. There are instances of taking on the burdens of others. Does your storage room hold the belongings of another? Have you moved this burden from place to place waiting for them to come and get it? Does it make you angry? Does the story line of needing everyone in our life to be "okay" before we meet our own needs sound familiar? Everyone else will have to be safe or content before we can take care of our needs. This is a way of saying: "I need to wait on the happiness of others. When they are happy and content, then I won't have to wait to meet my needs." Problems continue to grow when we use this type of excuse-making. Our family members, friends, or our working groups most likely do not need our help or our advice. Yet we persist in trying to be "helpful". So we wait. For many of us we are also overweight. Take a moment to reflect on these questions. Remember, we can't fix anyone. We can only change ourselves.

We believe in our uniqueness. True enough, there will never be another you. However, we can't use our sense of uniqueness as a way to avoid completing certain developmental tasks or facing the reality of life. This is called terminal uniqueness. Mastodons of the ancient ages were unique and are now extinct. We have to be aware that holding on to our uniqueness can be lethal. This is a form of wait and it becomes weight. If we pull out the retro-spectroscope, we can examine recent history for examples of those who gave up their lives because of an over-exaggerated sense of ability and an underestimated sense of reality.

# Why You Can't Have Your Cake & Eat It, Too

This is the Mount Everest experience. We all do it at one time or another. We ignore or pretend that our weight increase isn't harmful. We deny the significance of our symptoms. We may even form a club of other unique ones to bolster our position. After all, there is safety in numbers. We ignore our family genetics and nullify the effect of heredity on diabetes or heart events. We may be cavalier about the effect of research and believe there will be a cure before sickness comes to visit us. Or we may go the other way, sowing "wild oats" into the effects of chronic illness. We play "chicken" with our genetics, diet, and physiology. Those who died on the mountain are like those of us who weight/wait to excess. We ignore the obvious. Therefore, a huge price is exacted from us. The mountain experience exacted a huge price from those adventurers, and some very talented people died. Others were left to recover with some disfiguring injuries. Likewise some of us may die from the effects of our diseases. Others will be left to endure a life missing some important body parts like kidneys, eyesight, or lower legs. Mother Nature may just have the final say.

For a few moments, please contemplate some of these questions. This section has other questions you may wish to revisit in an examination of your belief systems. Contemplate how you resist this suggestion.

How do you experience waiting?

How much responsibility do you carry on your shoulders?

# Why You Can't Have Your Cake & Eat It, Too

What about the weight of history?

How do you clear the way?

When do you like to change?

What does personal responsibility mean to you?

# Why You Can't Have Your Cake & Eat It, Too

## The Challenge of Nutritional Mythology

Getting into the process described here will challenge much of what you have read and most of what you believe. Undoubtedly, much of what you have learned will be challenged as well. The old standard of "Eat less, exercise, and use some will power" just doesn't work. Beliefs in limiting portion size, recycling eating patterns, and the demands of exercising have weighed us down with more rules. It is an ongoing metabolic and mental gridlock. These forms of eating behaviors, nutritional mythologies, and other well-intentioned nutritional belief systems have become entrenched in our thinking. Even as they prove to be ineffective in controlling any weight-related consequences or health concerns we continue to obey them...

The challenge to our effort will be overcoming the formidable nutritional mythologies of our time. These mythologies are the food pyramid, portion control, calorie counting, and exercise as a means to attain ideal body size and/or health. A recent newcomer in nutritional mythology is the glycemic index. The food pyramid myth is deeply entrenched in our collective mind. It is a fundamental part of nutrition theory and is taught in medical and nursing schools alike. It is also taught to personal trainers. The so-called helping culture is resplendent with food pyramid, portion control, exercise, and glycemic mythology. It makes good fiction, and very poor science.

Would it come as a surprise to learn that the food pyramid has absolutely nothing to do with human physiology? It also has nothing to do with science. The food pyramid has everything to do with the physiology of the marketplace and the politics of food endorsement. In its early days of development politicians were warned that the food pyramid could create a public health disaster. The policy-makers in Washington told the scientists to make the science work to fit the food pyramid. This is the grand pyramid scheme.

The food industry has a huge economic investment in its survival, not yours. That is its purpose. The food pyramid represents a piece of the economic pie. If you look at its shape, you see pie all over it. Powerful lobbyists made sure every company they represented got a piece of the economic pie. Endorsement by the government was just the ice cream on top of that pie. When Congress held hearings on nutrition over 50 years ago, they had established the food pyramid first. They then went to the scientific community and asked them to validate it. The scientific community warned that America could not afford to be the nutritional guinea pigs for this effort. By this time the food industry was involved and the game was on.

The food pyramid system is responsible for the bankruptcy of public health. It is a formula for disaster. It has nothing to do with the way the human body functions. Nothing. Government agencies use the food pyramid for their so-called feeding programs. Is it any wonder that our Native Peoples are threatened with diabetes statistically more than any other group? It would seem that Washington never had a treaty with these indigenous people. They just continued the slaughter with diet and geographical changes.

Food makers have been very successful. They introduce lots of new and interesting choices to the market every day. It is difficult to come up with the number of new items introduced each year. Food labeling has become more creative and more sinister than a mystery novel. The FDA recently threw their hands up, saying the consumer was on his own when it came to interpreting labels. It seems the contents label has become a selling point for those looking for low-carb, low-fat, or low-salt items. Values are inflated or deflated to suit the whim of the market forces.

Since the inception of the food pyramid our obesity rates have doubled and now include youngsters. Diseases that afflicted adults are now impacting adolescents. Health insurance benefits are constantly being reduced. The chronic diseases are being under-covered, leaving the cost of prescriptions to the patient. These types of out-of-pocket expenses promote the profits of the drug companies, who no longer have to negotiate with insurers for coverage. One is forced to conclude that the drug and food companies are invested in keeping us sick. This will change only when people of good faith are invested in integrity. For the future we have economic shortsightedness, blinding us to the destruction of the public's health.

At present the food industry, public health officials, nutritionists, and lobbyists are working on a revision of the food pyramid mythology. A recent comment in the Wall Street Journal noted the new pyramid would be larger than the last one. In typical fashion, it will protect the market and ignore the public health.

Bear in mind that the old food pyramid has a caloric range of 2000-2500 calories a day. This is in direct opposition to their low-calorie myth. The portion sizes for the food pyramid as it now stands are huge. Fat intake is set at 65 to 80 grams a day. Carbohydrate intake is set at 300 to 375 grams a day. In caloric terms, these two items total 1500 to 2000 calories without the inclusion of protein. The food pyramid myth does not address the essential nutrient, protein, which is left out of their recommended daily allowances. We are left to our own invention when it comes to figuring out how much protein we need. The food pyramid mythology is counter to the grander myth of portion control/calorie-counting/exercise/glycemic-index ideology. It is no mystery how our society has become lost between the two concepts.

Even today with the burgeoning American waistline and increasing statistics on obesity-related chronic diseases, there is no sound of alarm. Somehow we still believe we are on top of things, and we can still handle it. It is gallows humor.

We don't need an outside invading army to destroy us. We are doing a great job of eating up our most precious resource - our health. The greatest pathogen is not a virus. It is the way we feed and nurture humanity. The food pyramid is the mythology of greed. It is disregard for the well-being of our cultures. Look to the example of the tobacco subsidy. Clearly this substance is the most toxic agent to human health, but it is still supported by our tax dollars through government hand-outs. The consequences of this misguided spending have created a health nightmare of death and economic drain, which is borne by all of us. Yes, we are all connected.

Portion control and calorie counting are as useless as the food pyramid in containing this approaching public health disaster. It just boggles the mind to see the corruptions that are supposed to be "balanced portions". We've all done it. Take 1000 calories of carbohydrates and call me in the morning. It happens with candy all the time. The portion control and calorie-counting theory has a false premise, -- that all calories or portions have the same value. In other words, there is no difference in the reactivity of protein, fat, or carbohydrate by the human metabolism.  The other fallacy of the calorie-counters and portion-controllers is that if the intake is kept low enough, then weight will be lost.  While in some instances there is weight loss,  problems arise when the loss is due to profound muscle depletion.  The furtherance of this notion is the advancement of the stomach-reducing surgery. It is the myth of the Emperor's New Clothes all over again.

There is a sad story coming out of this belief system, that  of people who continually harm themselves with restrictive starvation.  These are the bingers and purgers.  This is an equal-opportunity destroyer, affecting males as well as females.  Wrestling and ballet seem to have more than their share of these behaviors.   Following the bingeing is some kind of purgative attempt to undo the whole cycle.  Sometimes our suspicions should be aroused when we see or hear of young people dying at athletic events.

Exercise is used to force someone to change.  This is a way to stop waiting, true.  But what is a good time to get back into shape?.  It is not when someone is overweight, has high blood pressure, and has a displaced center of gravity.  Excess weight is tough on the delicate joints and spinal column, already  are under the significant strain of carrying excess weight.  It is much better to postpone rigorous exercise until the blood pressure and weight distribution have improved. Tendons holding muscle fiber to the bones can shred and snap if exercise is implemented unwisely or too soon.  Those who are taking lipid-lowering medication need to have special caution while going through exercise.  Tendons and ligaments can be weakened by these medications. Cautions need to be observed to prevent these types of injuries.

Exercise is also thought to be useful in spot reduction. A specific body part, it is believed, could be made smaller by repeated exercises done to that part. Most of us who have tried this technique will be able to draw the same conclusion. It doesn't work. This is an example of a collective myth, another false premise. This is the premise that calories "in" must the less than those expended for weight loss. The other false premise is that one can exercise to lose weight. It is just not true. There are many conditions that need to be aligned metabolically to obtain fat loss, which is different from weight loss. Here is the fact: a pound of fat is worth 3500 calories. That means, by the "calories-expended" theory one would have to do 3500 calories worth of physical work to obtain one pound of loss. This amount of work cannot be completed in one day. If it is done over a year's time, it is quickly undone by inappropriate feeding techniques.

The idea of portion control and exercise has created its own life and spun hopelessly out of control. Many folks who have tried portion control and/or exercise will tell you how it didn't work in attaining an ideal body size or ideal health. They will tell you how many times they were told by their health professionals to push back and exercise more. The health establishment is taught the food pyramid and calorie-counting plus exercise-more routine. Health professionals will prescribe this regime repeatedly. They will agree with their patient at some point that their obesity problem is hopeless. Instead of trying another approach or evaluating the individual's compliance, the surgical option is offered. Yes, what medicine can't fix, surgery will. Then the real sacrifice begins.

# Why You Can't Have Your Cake & Eat It, Too

This is the sacrifice of money, of malnutrition, and of morbidity.   This is the mythology of portion control which goes like this: controlling portion size will provide weight loss, a perfect body, a perfect life, perfect health and resolution of all life's problems.

Mythologies are stories.  They exist to help people understand the unknown qualities of life.  Sometimes they provide a small truth or carry a spiritual axiom.  They help explain why things happen as they do from a mythic realm.  They may teach a cultural belief system and make it seem more real.  Today the myths we see are used to bolster commerce.  They are not about health or truth.

I want to stress here that the medical establishment, the nutritional establishment, and the public all believe their myths. They have created an illusion.  It is possible that it will be true, but what if it weren't?  Are we willing to gamble that altering the size of the stomach or bypassing it altogether will solve the obesity problem?   In my practice I have seen substantial weight regained after stomach-altering surgery. The first postoperative year is the pink cloud.  Then life shows up.  I have heard the ways people get even or justify what they do, stomach-staple or not.  I have seen the malnutrition and kidney stones that result from the poor absorption taking from the gut.  I have heard about the intestinal gas, vomiting, and explosive diarrhea.

 Desperation is a subtle temptation.   It can lead us into chaos or it can lead us into challenge.  Recently there have been some developments in human nutritional research.  They have been discounted and discredited because of the economic and political consequences.

# Why You Can't Have Your Cake & Eat It, Too

Challenging this nutritional status quo reminds me of the story of the Emperor's New Clothes.  There are many parallels in this story.   We have a very self-absorbed emperor.  He is preoccupied with his self-image and his own comfort.  He is blinded to the reality of thieves masquerading as tailors. The Emperor needed to believe he was buying the only garment of its kind, one that would give him special advantages.  The main selling point was exclusivity. The Emperor took the bait and was soon wearing a suit of very expensive invisible clothes. All of the court, his trusted advisors, and the town bought into the concept of the Emperor's New Clothes.   It took just one person, a small child, to see the situation for what it was.

The commonly-held nutritional belief systems began as a way to explain health concepts.  Each culture will have a food or nutrient that conveys certain qualities to the user.  These qualities may be real or they may be imaginary.  An example of this is chicken soup.  As time passed, it became easy to manipulate the marketplace by using these nutritional belief systems.  Someone will create the special advantage myth and assign it to a nutrient.  This works even better if they write a book.  Government-endorsed feeding programs are based on the food pyramid, itself a perversion of human nutritional needs.  We all believe it.  We are afraid to challenge it because we don't want to cause undue distraction.  We don't want to embarrass the Emperor.

Are we not being stripped of our health and economic power? Let us remember how pension plans have been raided by greed.  It doesn't take too much of a stretch to see how our health has been raided by greed.  We are going to be responsible for the problem.  We must be. That is the only way we can be a part of the solution. We don't need another war on obesity. War is the wrong metaphor. We need to change the way we relate to the elements in nutrition. We need to change our belief systems. Human physiology is in a constant state of change. Our nutritional fairy tales lead us to believe we can outrun our biology. Our food fables give us The Emperor's New Clothes.

Each one of us is different. We react differently at different times to nutrients. This dynamic changes and is based on genetics. Think of these changes as being like the changes we experience with our eyesight or hair color.

## Making Resolutions

Making a resolution is a firm determination to take a specific course of action. Sometimes we confuse the determination with the result we are seeking. For example, we may resolve to take more vacations. We may even mark certain days off on our calendar. We search the Internet for airfares and flight schedules. Perhaps we select a destination. Now comes the hard part. Perhaps we have to request the time off if we are employed. Most of us will need a fair amount of money to take a vacation. We will need to pay for all the household expenses while we are way plus all of the expenses incurred on the trip. Sometimes we need to rent a car or to reserve a hotel room. All these activities are involved in planning ahead, in making preparations. This is work.

So what can we conclude? That making a resolution to do something requires work. which may involve planning, making phone calls, saving money, packing, and taking time off from work.    The process of resolving to do something is very different from the process of doing the resolution.

So what has this to do with getting healthy?  What has all of this to do with attaining an ideal body weight?  One of the things I hear frequently especially on January first is: "I am going to lose weight!  I really mean it this time!"  The list of reasons to do this may include some of the following:

- My daughter is getting married

- My high school reunion is this summer

- I don't like the way I look in the holiday pictures

- My doctor has been telling me to get the weight off

- My holiday eating and drinking is out of control

- XXL is my size! How did this happen?

These are the kind of reasons that lead us to resolve to lose weight/wait.  The health consequences associated with one's weight are rarely considered in the making of resolutions.  It would seem we are resolved to look good in front of our friends and family.

Soon the foundations of our resolve begin to crumble. Afflicted with weight and wait, we get cold feet. This is going to require deprivation!  It means work!  It takes time!

Then the justifications start to grow.  Could it be because of our lack of money?  Well, as soon as the anticipated tax refund comes in, then we will get the necessary help.  What about that an anticipated trip? Surely, we can't diet while away

## Why You Can't Have Your Cake & Eat It, Too

on a trip.   And then there are the upcoming holidays, - Valentine's Day, Easter,  St. Patrick's Day, and don't forget about your birthday.    Before we know it, half the year is gone.    The high school reunion is looming large on the horizon.  The tax refund has been used to pay for credit card balances left over from the holidays.

By this time it is June.  For some of us, we are already buying Christmas gifts.  Soon the end-of-the-year planning is in full swing.  As we look back over the year, we realize we didn't go to the reunion.  We may remember how we struggled to find the right dress or suit to wear to our daughter's wedding. There were countless essays constructed in our mind to explain why we were avoiding some important life events. Sometimes we would go for weeks in starvation to the feast for the weekends.

Time does seem to fly at all levels.   It flies when we are having fun, and it flies when we are procrastinating.   Time seems to evaporate in proportion to the amount of delay we establish in securing our future goals.   The more delay or wait we apply to our resolutions, the speedier is its flight.   "This time it will be different" is the language of resistance.  "If only" is the language of missed opportunity.   In a word, we are constantly living in he past or the future.  Let us resolve to live in the moment and to be curious with the process of change.

In an interesting way, making resolutions is like listing our resistances.  Look at the to-do lists!  They become the events that almost never get done.  Perhaps on New Year's Day it would be better to make a list of New Year's Resistances, so we would have a clear view of the things we have no intention of doing.  Yet paradoxically we long to do them.

# Why You Can't Have Your Cake & Eat It, Too

## Acceptance

Trying to get it back the way it was is impossible. This may come as a shock, but it is true. Our physiologic body is changing all the time. As hard as we try, it is impossible to push that reverse button. The body of our experiences deepens our wisdom and our faith. Learning to cope with the body you have now is a very tall order indeed, virtually a top-secret expedition into a foreign country. Then just as one mystery gets solved, another appears. One of my favorite quotes attributed to Bette Davis is "That which does not kill me makes me stronger". The plan just got bigger, and we lost the map.

In our attempts to impose control on our health woes, we often go out of control. There is a specific natural order to the way your physiology functions today. Much of that can be interpreted to you in meaningful ways. Powerful techniques will be presented to you that will be instrumental in your journey to health. Yielding to the processes showing up in your health picture will give us direction. There is an order in the natural process of creating health and in creating disease. Working with this natural progression we can regain what was lost: health, well being, and an ideal body weight. You do have a choice.

Having said all of that high-minded rhetoric, what does it all mean? It is one thing to say, and quite another to put into real-time practice. Sometimes a well-placed story will be of help. Let's start here. Let us just say one day you discover that your arms aren't as strong as they used to be. In fact, you notice that you can raise your arms up to your head, but they become tired in a very short period. This means you cannot arrange your hair just the way you would like. You also notice your arms don't have very much strength or power in terms of lifting. In fact, you are feeling quite helpless and defenseless.

Your first question is likely to be "How could this happen?". Many theories come to mind such as "If you don't use it you lose it." This thinking brings you to conclude that years of neglect and disuse have caused your muscles to become weak. Another idea might be "All older adults get weak muscles, so what is the use anyway?" Sometimes we may blame our weak arm muscles on unavoidable genetic flaws. Other popular concepts for understanding your weak arms might be to go to the library, the health food store, or the doctor in your quest for answers. In the meantime, your muscles in your arms are still weak. All of this searching for "why" has not changed this fact.

In the drama to understand why one has weak arm muscles, what about instituting a little elbow grease to address the problem? This means accepting your weak arm muscles as they are and taking action to correct the situation. So, for a beginning you set up a plan, such as: Four days a week for the next four weeks you decide to lift four-pound weights for four repetitions. Then your brain kicks in and tells you this is going way too slow. It's not worth it. Acceptance is thrown out the door. Somewhere in your gut a little voice reminds you how important your arms are, and how much you need them. Slowly the seeds of agreement begin to flow into your brain. Getting back to your plan, you decide to implement it. Additionally at the end of the first four weeks you are going to increase your repetitions to two sets of four repetitions.

# Why You Can't Have Your Cake & Eat It, Too

Months later you notice you can brush your teeth and arrange your hair with ease. Ah.

Acceptance is not resignation. Acceptance is wide-open recognition. As you begin to recognize your situation, it will then require action from you. When we have little children in a swimming pool we know we have to watch them constantly. This is acceptance. We may attach life vests to them while we are teaching them to swim. This is a plan. Once we teach them how to swim, we still watch them. This is acceptance. Part of teaching them how to swim is teaching them ways to be safe in water, such as "Never swim alone." This is the plan. Always we remind them where the steps are in the pool so they can rest when they are tired. This is acceptance.

We would never blame them for being tired or slow to progress. We would be patient while they learned little by little how to swim for longer times, and learn various swimming techniques. There would be praise for the smallest accomplishment. As they learned how to swim without the "floaties," they would know you were watching every stroke. You encourage them to go to the steps if they get tired, and they make steady progress. This achievement is made possible because as a parent you accepted that your child needed to be taught how to swim.

Accepting our responsibility as parents causes us to wear many hats. At some point action is required of us. Once you have determined that your child cannot swim, then it is up to you to implement a strategy that will yield a swimming child. Comparing your child to someone else's child does not produce a swimmer. Ignoring your child's need to swim will not produce a swimmer. Postponing your child's swimming lessons until a more convenient time will not produce a swimmer. Acceptance requires something of us. It requires action. Acceptance without action is just more delay. Wait.

From this example it is easy to see how impatient we are with ourselves. We can see how we compare ourselves to others. We may even recognize how we put off doing something today until some time in the future, when we get around to it. We may judge ourselves harshly. This is not acceptance. These are ways we distract ourselves from seeing the way we are in the world right now. We may even recite all of the facts we believe to be true as arguments to displace our personal responsibility for what is going on with our health. This is blame. It is not acceptance. It is weight and wait. The opposite of acceptance is resistance.

Sometimes by looking at what something is not; we can easily see it for what it is. Acceptance asks us to do something now. Not later.

**The Big Mystery**

Many of your medical mysteries can be solved. Our limited perceptions can be expanded. Opening the treasure chest of knowledge will require a key. All of this is a highly individual process. One strategy does not fit all. While it is true how different we are, we are different each and every day. Interpreting your particular medical mystery in a way that matters to you is the key. Hopefully this key will resonate in you, empowering you to grow in your changing dynamics. How often I hear "I know what to do, so why does this happen?" In that conversation are a couple of interesting inner contradictions.  One of those contradictions is the need to believe we know what to do.

How is it that we profess to know what to do and don't do it? It is what we know we know? Then what we know we don't know?  Then we know what we know, but don't know what we don't know.  Still more interesting is the stuff we don't want to know.  When we are presented with some new information, it gets discounted when we say, "Oh, that doesn't apply to me". There are many ways to dismiss and discount new truths. Remember you are on an expedition into the foreign territory of your changing body.  You can't afford to use the old stories to help you read the map.  The family myths about health and nutrition are based on superstition.  The marketplace is superstition-driven.

These new health paradigms presented to you aren't new. They go along with the human body's subtle energies of metabolic regulation. Keep a beginner's heart as you learn.

We are conflicted by the belief that we know what to do but don't know why "this" is happening to us. If we could know why, then all would be solved.  We would then cooperate metabolically speaking, of course, with whatever the Universe would decide.   If you know what, then you should know why we reason.

The hope is after reading these pages and interacting with the exercises you will know what you don't know.  You will understand why you have become glucose-intolerant. You might even understand how your body became over-fat. Your intolerance to glucose and the insulin reaction with its cascade of physical complaints will be clear to you.  Lastly, you will be presented with ongoing complementary strategies that will support your intent to become healthy.

"Becoming healthy" will have a different viewpoint for each person.  Some will simply need to lose stored body fat.  Some will require blood sugar control.  Others will need to improve their blood pressure management.  Indigestion, fluid retention, and sleep apnea may also be a part of the landscape, physically speaking.  Finding the target for your strategic plan may include all the problems listed plus some others.  However we work it, we will constantly be checking in with your body as to how it manages its insulin reserves and its energy reserves.  Superstitions about nutrition will not work.

## Standing in Line - the Test of Patience

Imagine you are going to the movies, to  the  opening night of a first-rate performance.   After parking the car, we arrive at the marquee to find a line forming in front of the theater.  We would like to grumble, but we decide to get in line.  We look at the starting time for our movie and we glance at our watch.  We say to ourselves, "It won't be too much longer, so let's wait."  Others begin to arrive and the line  grows longer.  We congratulate ourselves for arriving early and having a spot in the line so close to the door.  We have yet to purchase our tickets, yet we wait.

Our waiting is uncomfortable.  We are tired of standing, but we all agree it will be worth it.  This is going to be a great movie!!  Suddenly, we see a large black limousine pull up to the curb in front of the theater.  Out of it emerges some kind of celebrity.  She is all dressed up in the fashion of the moment.  Additionally, she is attended by a large contingent of bodyguards. There is also an entourage. They make their way to the front of the line. As they approach the ticket taker, there is the beginning of a commotion. Their spokesperson insists they are expecting to get in the door without paying for a ticket. They are also expecting to get in first because of their special importance. They stress the expectation of not having to wait with the rest of the line.

The ticket taker informs the bodyguards, the celebrity, and the entourage that they have no special privileges. They are further informed that they have to get in line and wait just like everyone else. As you can imagine, this does not go over well. The entourage demands to see the manager. The manager arrives.

Soon the combatants square up. The manager informs the interested entourage that they are not getting in before those of us who are in line. She tells them that they have to wait just like everyone else. It seems she will not be bribed.

Undaunted by the manager of the theatre, the entourage pushes forward. They continue to move forward, regardless of the denials of the manager and the ticket taker. Tempers begin to heat up. Words are exchanged. Soon the security team is summoned. The police may be called. More bodyguards spill out of the limousine. Perhaps the fire department of the local municipality is summoned. The local police department reinforces the security measures taken by the theatre. It becomes apparent that the groups are at a stand-off. The celebrity is standing out on the sidewalk, surrounded by her entourage, and all are surrounded by the strong forces of the local municipalities. This is resistance, is it not?

# Why You Can't Have Your Cake & Eat It, Too

Meanwhile back at the line, we are waiting.  Just the waiting is irritating on its own merit.  To make matters even more interesting, we are becoming hot and thirsty.  Impatient to get into the theater, we are getting angry.  Opinions are bandied about.  Some of us say, "Oh, just let them in.  Get this thing over so we can get in." Others will say, "Oh, no. They need to wait just like the rest of us. Who do they think they are?" We may have loud discussions.  As a group, we are getting irritated for a variety of reasons.  We have tried to play by the rules and wait our turn.  It would seem the theater and the conflict should be easy to settle.  With the police presence, it would seem that resolution is near.  Yet, we wait.

To compound our irritation and misery we learn we have missed the start of our first-run movie.  Our disappointment swells into anger.  We had a few of our own expectations and they are increasing our irritation.  Standing in line has a few unspoken rules.  One of them is that the person closest to the door gets in first.  Another unspoken rule is that latecomers should have to wait just like everyone else, bribery not included.   Most of the time latecomers will go to the end of the line.  All of us have seen how individuals will "save" places in the line for their friends.  As irritating as this practice is, most of us will look the other way.

In our story we are looking at a social situation that has a symbolic relationship to waiting and weight.  There is force, resistance, preferential treatment, more force, and irritation. The line is not moving into the theater.  The security team is holding the entourage back at the door.  The police are forming a staging area.  We could be in the middle of a full-scale riot.  Tempers are heating up.  Words are being exchanged between all of the parties.   Laws may be broken. And, we are still waiting.

We all seem to understand the laws of supply and demand, an important force in commerce.   Much work goes into the preparation required to open a theater.   It is a business just like any other.   Workers are hired.   Supplies are bought. Contracts are made with the big moviemakers.   A building is designed to contain all of this magic.   It is a work of art.   This all costs a lot of money.   Customers supply this business with their money.   They come into the theater to buy tickets, food, and drink.   Customers are the lifeblood of commerce.   They are supplying it with life-sustaining energy.

In our story, our customers are kept waiting.   Some of them may leave to go to another venue.   Some of them may be so irritated they will vow never to go to another movie.   The entourage is still arguing their case of importance.   They are on their cell phones trying to get the news media to show up with cameras and lights.   The management, security teams, and local law enforcement have all performed their functions as they were trained to do.   They have resisted the incursion of a celebrity, her entourage, and her bodyguards.   The media are now here, bringing in cameras and lights.

The sidewalk is clogged.   There is more irritation.   There is more resistance.   There is pressure.   There is need.   Our theater is under siege.   Eventually this event takes place every day.   It used to happen twice a week.   The frequency increases the consequences.   Customers figure out soon enough that they will have to go elsewhere.   If there is even a hint of a disturbance, customers go somewhere else.   Slowly, this theater begins to lose its employees.   Maybe they can no longer pay their bills.  The customers have become sensitized to this type of disturbance.  It doesn't take long for the doors to close.  Soon many locations experience this phenomenon of waiting and resistance.  It is a repeating story of abundance and extinction.

Imagine the business or theater as a cell in the body.  Perhaps imagine the theater is the body.  The celebrity is playing the role of carbohydrates.  Her bodyguards get the job of representing insulin.  The entourage is just more carbohydrates and more insulin.  The ticket taker, manager, and security teams are the resistance of the body. The presence of the media symbolizes the signs and symptoms created by insulin resistance.  The fire department is a symbol for many of the interventions created to change this dynamic. The waiting lines of customers represent protein, fat, and water.  They are the wait and the weight.

Commerce is a very simple process.  A supply of consumers returning for the expected good service at a business venue is something a viable enterprise wants to nurture.  It acts like a magnet.  Whether one is a worker, an owner, or a customer, we place value in the nourishment of commerce.  And yet, there is a little more to add to this story.

Those of us who stood by in lines, waiting patiently for our turn,  have the opportunity to express our will.  But, we didn't. We let someone else do it.  Had we gotten involved in the sidewalk dynamic, change might have occurred with less drama, less resistance.  Often when we find ourselves in this situation, we become that "silent majority."  We may roll our eyes, and pretend we are somewhere else.  We may be concerned about drawing attention to ourselves.  We remained silent and simmering. To be effective in this type of situation, one has to get involved. This might mean being willing to take the responsibility for the change that needs to happen.

In the symbolic story we saw how much resistance the theatre had to apply to the dynamic at the front door. How much stronger the position of the theater would be if those of us in line expressed our unified will. Our celebrity exists because of a magnetic attraction we have for stardom. There are many "what-ifs" here, but imagine the impact of the unity of our collective voices. What if we let the theater know about our concerns? What if we addressed the celebrity directly? What if we had made known what our expectations were? Our impatience is irritation. Our desire is to go to see a movie, but we got sabotaged. This is a form of irritation. In groups there is often a delay in taking action until a leader can be identified. This is a part of the waiting this story is about.

It takes time for this story to unfold. In each one, there are many warning signs, which we choose to ignore. In the descriptions that follow there are interesting parallels to the waiting-in-line idea and insulin resistance. On one scale we observe how the idea of personal choice manifests in the development of irritations and blockages. On the physiologic scale these interactions create and relate to the same irritations and blockages.

Throughout all of time, story has been used to teach and to explain. The story presented here is an attempt to present in language the phenomenon of insulin resistance and obesity. Up until now, we have had little new common understanding about obesity and its related co-morbidities. This "waiting-in-line concept" is an idea that may resonate with many who have these issues or who are concerned about someone with insulin resistance.   Myth and fable have been used to teach and explain, but they have another purpose, to warn us so that if we so choose, we can outrun an unintended result.

## Waiting in Line or Weighting the Line

Going back to the line-crasher idea in our story, we can build the metaphor to make the point about insulin resistance. Typically the words "non-insulin-dependent diabetes" gives the perception that the pancreas is deficient or not producing enough insulin.   While it may be partially true, it is not the whole story.  In the line-crasher metaphor, glucose is the line-crasher and insulin is its burly bodyguard pushing into the cell. As the cell resists the push of the insulin bodyguard, the pancreas readily supplies more power in the form of more and more insulin bodyguards.   Imagine a big forward line of glucose with its burly insulin bodyguards.   The crowding, the pushing, the shoving is causing a pressure build-up in the vessels. Some of us may get high blood pressure.  The cells in the blood vessels that are charged with the duty of maintaining blood pressure cannot perform correctly because of the build-up of glucose and insulin.  They cannot expand and contract, for instance, because of the compressed vascular environment.  As the blood pressure begins to build, as we feel miserable, we will eat to keep going.  Typically this means more carbohydrates.  Then just as things get bad, they get worse!  The insulin production is stimulated again and again by more incoming glucose.  Wave after wave of insulin tries to move the blood sugar out of the blood and into the cell.   This sets the stage for glucose toxicity and insulin resistance. With the over-secretion of insulin we now have

# Why You Can't Have Your Cake & Eat It, Too

"Code Red" conditions in the body. This is the beginning of Metabolic Syndrome X. This syndrome is characterized by too much insulin, too much blood glucose, and the resistance of the body to those elements.

Now we have too many line-crashers and too many bodyguards! So what happens next? The security force gets called. The metaphor expands as the security forces get into the fray. This is the beginning of resistance. For our purposes, this is insulin resistance. So in real time, real life, the body goes into hyper-alert. Imagine the internal stress created by this type of resistance. There is an irritation present between the security guards and the burly bodyguards. They may argue even fight. Remember, this is cellular resistance to insulin and glucose.

The development of the internal resistance cycle has an auto-immune-like response. This is like an allergy. The release of cortisol in response to the stress of high blood sugar will develop. This is called a volume overload. The amazing human body, in an attempt to downgrade the glucose toxicity, will release adrenalin-like hormones to help. To make matters more interesting, more insulin will be created as well. The helper mechanism compounds the cellular disorder. It is at this point the kidneys react by selecting the sodium-linked fluids for retention. Fluid retention is a common complaint. Try to remember that your body is trying to protect its vital, life-supporting organs. It will do this with the retention of fluid around these areas. This fluid retention will expand to all areas of the body. So when your toes and fingers get puffy, you know the fluid has reached the last place for it to go.

# Why You Can't Have Your Cake & Eat It, Too

Back at the queue there is another development.  Let us say our line has formed at the movie.  We have the insulin body-guards escorting its celebrity to the front.  We have the additional security forces attempting to create order.  We have the line waiting.   Waiting is irritating on its own!!   Just as in commerce, when customers cannot get goods or services from a business, the business goes bankrupt.  The customers cannot buy a ticket to see the movie.  They cannot enter the theatre to buy consumables.  The commerce is disrupted.

So too, do we have a physiologic disruption.  Nutrients are held up waiting in line.  Waiting for resolution of the argument at the door of our theatre may take hours or days.  Our customers may go elsewhere.  The resistance is costing more and more.   The net effect is our theatre goes out of business, and people lose their jobs.  The market is cut off and there is isolation from the business world.   This metaphor can be used to explain insulin resistance and its myriad symptoms.  It is devastating to go out of business, to endure cutbacks in profits, to lose one's standing in the economic community, and lose employees.  This picture takes place in our body as it experiences insulin resistance.

Here we have a large willing pool of consumers (fat and protein) desiring to use our service (cell), but they can't get in the door (insulin resistance).  Water is held back.  The defensive strategies performed by the administration (body) are enacted too late, too little, or too much.  These reactions create calculated consequences.  A sense of weight is felt.  There is waiting.  This is the beginning of a breakdown in communication between the business (cell) and the customer (nutrients and water), and it is the beginning of going-out-of-business.  This economic peril, or loss of health,  parallels the symptoms and afflictions experienced by chronic insulin resistance.

When we begin to eat something, for the most part we are not intending to get over-fat.  It is not our intention to lose our eyesight, toes, or kidneys by what we eat.  We want to be a part of life, not a particle of life.  We want to keep our body working and all in one piece.  Our theater found out too late the cost of being overrun by non-paying brutish customers.  They lost everything.   Had they acted sooner with swift effective planning, the results might have been different.  This is what we must do to save ourselves.  We cannot wait.  It is weight.

## The Conflict Rages

Many nutritional theorists of our time, such as Suzanne Sommers, Dr. Atkins, Dr. Weil, and Dr. Phil, have created some complex food rules. The commercial diet plans, of which there are legion, have done a good job of amassing fortunes on the miseries of many, doing direct marketing of products. It is in their best interest to keep us eating mystery food. Books by the carload have been written for us "carbohydrate addicts with blood types in the zone needing sugar busting." It is a highly polarizing issue.  The nutritional tri-fecta is about portion control, calorie counting, and exercise. These are the big three myths of weight management. Will power is also suggested as a factor in weight management.  What does a balanced healthy diet mean after all? Is it the food pyramid? Is it fiber? Is it fat free?

This thinking is deeply engrained in our culture on all levels. Medicine, nursing, and nutritionists for the most part embrace this thinking as well.  If portion control, calorie counting, and exercise don't work, then there is surgery.

The food pyramid is a part of the collective mind.  It was created and endorsed by the government.  The FDA led the way for this food scheme with a crafted plan to give favoritism to the food industry.  Knowing that no particular food could be singled out for limitation or exclusion, the broad food pyramid was devised, produced and directed by powerful food lobbyists.  We all remember the persecution by food companies of those hapless celebrities who have voiced any negative views about it.  Agriculture is big business.  We need business, and business needs us.  People working in these industries are just as affected by insulin resistance as everyone else.  Like the Great Pyramids of Egypt, the food pyramid is archaic.

Remember the groups meeting in Washington to revise and improve the food pyramid? These groups will consist of the self-interested.  They will dress it up in new colors, and make it more difficult for anyone to understand.  Remember, they are doing this complex food strategy under the old myth: it is for our own good.  The pyramid is a political solution to the distribution of food and the wealth flowing from those channels.  It is a pyramid scheme of the highest order.  We have wrongly assumed that the government would place the highest scientific minds in charge of the food guide pyramid.  Science is nowhere to be found in the creation or development of this complex scheme.  It is a little-known fact that scientists warned the government about the food pyramid when it was first developed in the 1980's.  The scientific community warned the Senate that they were gambling with the public health.  Money has a louder voice.

## Why You Can't Have Your Cake & Eat It, Too

Then there is the American Diabetic Association.  They are aligned with the food pyramid ideology.  The ADA has trained countless dietitians and diabetics on management of their diets.  This organization is supported by the food and drug industry.  From its results, it would appear they have no interest in getting people well.  Diabetics who have been exposed to the traditional ADA plan are consuming an average of 200 to 300 grams of carbohydrates a day, if not more.  Their blood sugars, weight, and dire health consequences are the direct result of the "balanced diet and medicine" the plan proposes.  Many diabetics consume more than these carbohydrate guidelines.  The progression of the disease of insulin resistance is not halted or controlled with this plan.  As we watch these populations age, we can see steady deterioration.  As healing professionals, our intention is to do no harm.  Yet the ADA continues to teach the same old concept: eat lots of carbohydrates and take lots of drugs to manage blood sugar.  It is a win-win for the drug companies and the food industry.

Complicating this situation is the limited training the newly diagnosed diabetic individual is able to obtain.  Insurance will not pay for nutritional counseling on an ongoing basis.  Most of the time if this service is allowed, it is for one time only. It will not be individualized or culture-sensitive.  These services will be done in large groups with little time for support or inquiry.  Then one is left to one's own diet design.  Slowly or quickly the old portion-control calorie-restricted ideology will rear its ugly head. Reinforced by the culture of consumerism, cheered on by the drug companies, our diabetic will struggle in vain to control her blood sugars or weight. Our diabetics will endure countless complications and admonishments.   The ADA guidelines allow for the blood sugar to be maintained at

# Why You Can't Have Your Cake & Eat It, Too

180 mg/dL.  This 'acceptable level for treatment' is destructive to the tissues.  This blood sugar environment begins the slow descent into the hell of chronic debilitating disease. It is hell for the diabetic, but heaven to big business.

At this time, the health insurance industry would prefer to pay for Bariatric surgery than to teach individuals how to nourish themselves appropriately.  Lately the health insurers have put a halt to paying for these surgeries due to the high cost involved, due in part to the complex management of the morbidly obese patient.  Then there are the complications following the surgery that no one wants to talk about.  The statistics following Bariatric surgery cover only the first thirty days.  If you don't keep score, then you don't have to know how the game is going.  Bariatric surgery is another medically unsupervised scheme for the patient to avoid taking responsibility for his or her own condition.

65% of our country is dangerously obese as of the year 2003. In 2001 the JAMA calculated the obese population to be at 61%.  This is a staggering mathematical progression. Two-thirds of this country's people are insulin resistant.  This is an epidemic in waiting/weighting.   People are going to require tremendous medical and economic resources for their care. The burden to the family and the country will be enormous. The level of obesity denial is evidenced by the ridiculous adaptations  we see on this issue.   Motorized chairs, larger coffins, and bigger airline seats. Is anyone listening?

Astonishing as it is, even in the face of increasing human obesity, calorie-counting, portion control, and exercise are still endorsed by most credible medical practitioners. The dietary professionals will also take this position. Dismissing the theory of insulin resistance and its relevance in the creation of disease, they will exhort their clients to cut back a little more. Often exercise is implemented as the sure way to obtain the desired result.  One sees 300-pound individuals literally driving up their blood pressure and destroying their joints with vigorous exercise.  With the body carrying 120 extra pounds of fat, the center of gravity is off.  Losing one's balance and falling can be a serious problem.

This becomes a hopeless effort.  Many just give up.  It is hard to endure being hungry and the sense of failure the "calorie-counting, portion-controlling, exercise-more" culture has instilled in the collective mind.  This culture has a strong need to be right. Your difficulty with portion control, calorie counting, and exercise, they tell you, is about your lack of will.  Soon you believe that there is something lacking in you.  You have tried everything and nothing has worked.   I have seen patients who have totally lost hope in the ability to manage their own weight.  Often there are layers of belief systems operating at different levels.  All of these layers need to be peeled away to expose what an individual believes to be true for him or her.   This need to find solid ground nutritionally is the missing piece of the puzzle.  Solid ground is not arrogant, does not put on airs, and is not puffed up, to paraphrase some old wise words.  Assisting you to reach your desired goal is hard work.  Hearing you voice your heart's desire is very significant to this work.

Many times the theorist or practitioner will put his imprint on what you should weigh.  Often this "goal weight" is not attainable or even maintainable.   To make matters more difficult, you are not given a say in what it is you would like to do. Listening to the dreams of each one is important.  Often the answer is there.  It takes careful observation and listening with the heart to help change course, while on the journey to get healthy.   The road map is often there, but locked away in the glove box.   We will try to remove the resistances that block the way.  Let's live the dream and not the nightmare.

Previously mentioned is the proliferation of Bariatric surgeries done to the stomach to reduce its capacity to hold food.  The idea is to force someone to eat smaller portions.  The reduced stomach is not able to hold large quantities of food without causing vomiting and distention.  A band may be used around the stomach, or the stomach may be stapled to a smaller size.  The by-pass surgery is done to re-route the food from the stomach directly into the small intestine.  This will result in fast dumping of the stomach contents without the absorption of nutrients and calories.  In this scenario, the negative intended result from over-indulgence would be frequent loose stools, distention, or vomiting.   One would think this would be a significant deterrent.

Time and again I have seen this type of negative reinforcement fail.   Interviews with patients who have experienced failures with  Bariatric surgeries will describe how they overrode the surgery.  They used soft foods repeatedly.  These foods could be warm or cool, but they were smooth.  These foods slip pass the "ring" or the small pouch in the stomach.  Small pieces of soft chocolate candies, cake, and ice cream slide through the site.   In no time at all, they had regained all the weight they had initially lost, plus more.  Complicating this picture is  poor absorption from the gastro-intestinal tract.  This leads to malnutrition, kidney destruction, and osteoporosis.  If you were sick before, you really have something to talk about now.

# Why You Can't Have Your Cake & Eat It, Too

Bariatric surgery synthesizes all of the weight-loss myths. Deeply embedded in the collective mind of the popular culture is the myth of portion control, calorie counting, will power, and exercise as the way to obtain weight management. Often a person who is contemplating this type of surgery will go through numerous diet plans so they can demonstrate their futility. The reality is that the diet plan failed because it did not address the insulin resistance in the patient. Remember that most of the commercial diet plans are created around portion control and calorie counting. Yet the patient will take on this type of diet failure to show how hopeless their obesity is and what a failure they have become. The patient will become their body as an indication of their failure as a human being. They will say that they have tried portion control and it didn't work. They tried will power with the same result. They have exercised and didn't lose weight. Then surgeons have created a surgery in support of this myth. They believe that forced portion control with this surgery is the only way to help a hopelessly obese person, as does the patient by this time.

Physicians take a one-hour class in nutrition in medical school. Today this type of "short" classes are taken on-line. To suggest someone change the shape of someone else's stomach or intestine based on such limited exposure to nutrition is extraordinary.

Insulin resistance is the cause and the cure of our obesity epidemic. It is not a failure of the human being. It is conclusion based on a false information. It has persisted for many years based on its resistance to change its knowledge about human nutrition. The refusal to accept insulin resistance as the sole causative factor in obesity is about fear

-- fear about scarcity of work, product, and jobs. True enough, there will be many people crippled by obesity. If these people get healthy, chose food products differently, require less care, need less medicine, and become productive again, what will the businesses that have profited from this disease do?

Bill Maher made the following comment on his program about this public health problem. He said, "Stomach stapling is going to be as effective as gluing a cocaine addict's nostrils shut. They will find another way." Well, I might not approve of his comparison, but I think he raises a point. The stomach is not the problem in obesity. The nose is not the problem to the cocaine addict. What is on the inside has a way of showing up on the outside. The conflicted inner self has a way of mirroring itself on the external self. Add to that inner conflict fostered by the faulty nutritional belief systems. A perfect human being is transformed into unspeakable human suffering.

Suffering is something we do. Being is something we are.

**A Healing Thought**:

For the next few moments, consider your perfect inner self.

Breathe.

Connect your highest intention to your soul's highest purpose.

Rest your mind. Turn it to the off position. Get the censor to log off.

## Why You Can't Have Your Cake & Eat It, Too

Ground your physical being in the energy of the protective presence of the Universe.

Breathe.

You will solve your mysteries.  You will be well.

You will choose wisely, forgive everything, and accept this opportunity to heal.

Breathe.

You are good.  You are wise.  You are healing.

Hold that thought, and breathe.

# Why You Can't Have Your Cake & Eat It, Too

## The Collective Unconscious and the Mind of Our Culture

The cascading symptoms that flow from the disease of obesity are the focus of modern medical treatment. High blood pressure, reflux, fluid retention, irritable bowel, spastic colon – all of these are symptoms. Symptoms are the effects of something, but the root causes are rarely addressed.  If obesity is addressed, our health professional will say something like, "Just eat less and exercise". This is what I hear, again and again. It is impossible to figure out what needs to be done, even if we are willing to do it.  We are afraid to fail, so we don't even try!   Attempting to find and implement a lasting nutritional life-plan is often met with loud guffawing from our peers as they say, "Oh, there she/he goes again."

To further complicate the situation, close personal friends or a health professional will try to pull the rug out from under your effort.  They will throw up some very well-placed fears, like grenades intended to displace you.  This fear is usually directed to your "best interests".  Actually, this tactic is far removed from your best interest or best efforts, for many of these fear-based spin-doctors are simply trying to rain on your parade. It is like running into a tank while on a skateboard. The scene might play in many ways.  Sometimes there will be the use of comparison to derail you. You are told a story about someone who knew someone who did what you are doing and then.... their kidneys dropped out.  Occasionally there is judgment targeted your way, perhaps by someone pouncing on a technique you are implementing and torpedoing your rationale with some spin-doctoring nutritional mythology.  This might include some very frightening polysyllables you have never heard of.  One of my favorites in this category is 'free-radical'. Who wants a free radical living next door? Anti-oxidants, bio-flavinoids, micronutrients, and many more alien life forms are set out like armies to threaten your effort. This is a clever tactic used to make someone feel nutritionally inferior. Such an inferiority complex has many purposes. One purpose is to get us to buy more useless health food products or to eat tons of foods in order to provide us with these so-called vital nutrients. Another purpose is to instill fear of doing something dangerous or not "medically'" approved.

There are huge nutritional databases available in the bookstore. Anyone of us can purchase one of these food dictionaries. Look up the popular food myth of the moment and you will see for yourself how transparent these medi-informercials are. The moral of the story is that talk is cheap. Try not to take someone's pet cause-of-the- week personally. Don't assume they are right.

There are those who are more interested in being right about something than they are in supporting you. Little heed is given to the gravity of the disease processes at work in your particular situation. Often it is said, "The enemy of good is better". This has been the cause of all types of injustice from the beginning of time. Caution is advised when you hear the words, "This is for your own good." The reality of that statement is, "This is for my own good, not yours."

Some of the fear projectiles are found in the realm of tribal or collective belief systems. The dietary establishment will attempt to create a fear of getting cancer if fiber is not used in the diet. The reality of good bowel health requires lots of water and a little oil. The food pyramid tribe will attempt to create a fear of vitamin deficiency if any one of the food groups is omitted.   The medical establishment will use fear of organ destruction should high-protein diets be implemented. Working groups are just like our families in parroting something they happen to read in a popular magazine. They try to act like parents!

The family will have a specific nutritional belief system tailored to meet its needs. You may remember being told not to waste food.  Even if the food is not good for you, you will feel guilty about it sitting on the shelf getting old. The dietary culture will suggest that cancer will be caused by the lack of balance in the diet.   The exercise culture will attempt to create fear of loss of cardiac benefit or muscle meltdown if their guidelines are not followed.  They will further insist that calories-in must equal calories-out.  Again and again, this is about the need to be right and to get some kind of pay-off.  These fears are about them.  They are not  about you.  In fact, we have so much stuff to fear, we can't discern the real fear from the imaginary, political or commercial.

Many of these "they-say" remarks are going to be directed at you.  Here is where the subtle inner voice is going to start nudging you.  Remember to pay it heed.  There is no doubt or fear in that.  Try not to analyze or justify or compare what is going on with you to anyone else.  Simply ask yourself, "Does this item or situation truly nourish my soul?"  The eloquent William Shakespeare writes in the play Hamlet; "To thine own self be true".  In this there is no argument or judgment.

It sometimes defies logic to believe what we are told we should believe.  I have looked at some of these informational cascades, and found them to be inherently misguided.  We depend on information-gatherers to provide us with information. It takes a lot of time and money to locate good information, so we become dependent on the information culture to provide us with important research. We also come well-equipped with our cultural belief systems about many things. We will filter new information through these inherited belief patterns. Often we select information that parallels our cultural belief patterns.

What happens is that the information that is heard the most often and is said the loudest is assumed to be correct. All informational systems are not created equal. Some want you to buy something. Some want you to be afraid so you will buy something. Some will want you to avoid one thing and prefer something else, and (you guessed it) buy it. Other informational cascades will lead off with words like "This could happen, or that may happen, etc." These informational cascades are about fear. Fear drives demand for all kinds of things. It is at the nexus of commerce.

We live in the age of information, which should help us to be free, not fearful. In no time at all we are all thinking alike! The informational cascade that deals with weight management is inefficient because it is based on false information. This wrong-way information needs to be changed. One of the latest developments in this area is the glycemic index. It has as its premise that any particular food will react the same way in all people. This conclusion was based on studies of so called normal people. The sample group of "normals" fasted overnight. In the morning they were given food and blood values were drawn. From the results, a glycemic index was made.

# Why You Can't Have Your Cake & Eat It, Too

There are several problems with this glycemic index.  One is its application to the diabetic and other insulin-resistant individuals.  These classes of people are no longer "normal".  They are going to demonstrate huge variances in blood sugars and blood insulin levels in response to any food.  They will not fit the profile.  As such, the glycemic index cannot be used for the therapeutic diet.  Another problem with the glycemic index is the fact that this study was never replicated.  In other words, the study needs to be repeated over and over to see if the same results can be obtained.  This cannot be done because it is not possible.  What are "normal" volunteers after all?  We know that each one of us will react differently to caffeine or aspirin for instance.  How can we be expected to react the same way to the same food?

The glycemic index theory then spawned a huge food empire.  The nightmare continues to this day.

The thoughtful work of Robert Atkins, Gerald Reaven, and Jean Pierre Flatt has demonstrated that portion control, calorie-counting, and exercise have no effect on insulin resistance, which is an important development in our overweight populations.  Their work has also shown that fat loss is dependent on insulin resistance.  The other side of the coin, insulin resistance also contributes to fat gain. There is also an interesting parallel running with this type of resistance.  The word resistance implies a strong repelling force.  It is helpful to think of insulin resistance as an autoimmune process.  Insulin resistance takes place in the body.  Intellectual resistance takes place in the mind.  Refusal to accept change is resistance in the soul.  They go hand in hand.  Stubbornness is resistance.  This is a different look at the complexity of insulin resistance.

# Why You Can't Have Your Cake & Eat It, Too

Freethinking individuals unaffected by social pressures or economic gain can reverse the effects of wrong-way information cascades. In order to heal insulin resistance and obesity we need to talk about our belief systems and look at the fear these belief systems support. Then we can replace these old beliefs with good information based on science and the physiology of nutrition.

## Games We Play

We have tried food games, exercise games, and starvation games. Plugging in our worn-out cultural belief patterns will not work any more. Listing these numerous schemes is like counting the stars in the sky. Many times we fall back to portion control, calorie counting, and exercise. Some of us may try drugs, both over and under the counter, for appetite control. There is surgery to make the stomach conform to our will. We will discard the parts of us we don't like, hoping to rub the lamp and get three wishes. There may be some successes, but they are often short-lived. Insulin resistance doesn't go away. Our cultural biases reflect our collective resistances. Soon we return to our old ways. Go figure, yes, and there goes our figure!

The interesting thing about games is the rules. The games we play have the quality of fairness implied in the rulebook. Someone who is weak, simply by being clever can easily maneuver a strong player. This ability to be clever is rewarded by winning the game. Then in another round, the tables may be changed. So a strong technique may overpower someone with the same skill who may be physically weak.

# Why You Can't Have Your Cake & Eat It, Too

Some of the simple board games we play can be enjoyable to lose when we are playing with a child. In the life game, we don't have definable rules.  Our indefinable rules, the ones that govern the collective mind, are a part of our problem, and they require healing.  As long as we live in our expectations, create resentments, and exact revenge we will create countless aberrations in life-enhancing behavior. These are also known as justifications.  As long as we persist in portion control, calorie-counting, and exercise to manage insulin resistance we will continue to destroy our collective health and become overweight.

Each one of us needs to claim our personal authority from the almighty "They."  They are the collective drug companies, the government, the insurance industry, the food lobby, and the medical establishment.  Insulin resistance and intellectual resistance can be challenged with serious personal commitment. We need to look at the way we procrastinate, avoid, justify, stuff, and otherwise perpetuate our collective myth-driven obesity epidemic.  We need to start the engines, now.

Remember, you cannot have your cake and eat it too.

## Reference Points

Most of us have many nutritional guides lining our bookshelves at home.  When we discuss nutrition in social groups, it becomes a hotly-debated topic.  The constant seeking of opinions is a technique used to postpone taking effective action. It is a part of the wait/weight phenomenon. We all are experts; we can cite case after case to support our opinions, and we know someone who knows someone, et cetera.

All of the diet books in the bookstores help to create  much confusion.  I have also noticed an interesting trend regarding the popular theories these books generate.  Individuals are going to one-day seminars to become certified as facilitators for a particular weight management scheme.  They may have no other scientific study or internship with these concepts. Often I see these concepts get mingled, or jumbled, with the personality of the facilitator and her personal nutritional mythology.  In general, what I can say after reading many of these diet or nutrition books is that they focus on will power, calorie counting, portion control, exercise, and (gasp) the dreaded food pyramid.   It is nothing new - it just looks different.

In the instance of the "Atkins diet," I have yet to see it practiced twice the same way.   Most people who follow this plan focus on fat intake.  The fat emphasis, I believe, was Dr. Atkins' way of creating a new paradigm.  He was trying to go against the low-fat-high-carbohydrate-eating fad that has created the diseases of insulin resistance and obesity.   Fat does not create a demand for pancreatic insulin, thereby increasing fat oxidation. That means the fat gets burned up or used by the body.   The point of protein need is missed completely by most readers of his theory.  Protein is another nutrient that is vital to the human body. Like fat, it does not generate an insulin response, thereby increasing fat oxidation. Carbohydrates, on the other hand, generate an insulin response, which impedes fat oxidation.   This is what Dr. Atkins was trying to say, in my opinion.   The media, the collective information-gatherers, have distorted the "Atkins diet" into a bacon-consuming, half-and-half-guzzling stereotype.

Sometimes we choose a particular weight management scheme based on the look of the book cover. It attracts us, and imitation is the sincerest form of flattery. We are attracted to what we want to be. Perhaps we have a friend who tried a certain form of "diet." Her results are a good demonstration, so you try it. Success is a good attractor. However, the diet doesn't fit you and your physiology, so another tome hits the bookshelf at home. The supply is endless.

While values of personal responsibility are regarded highly as important, personal responsibility has little value in the creation of health. One place where our responsibility is abdicated is in our health care systems. Have you ever tried to read your health plan's manual or list or providers? Our healthcare delivery systems are overloaded (weight) with rules. Who is really taking care of us and bearing the responsibility for it? Who has the power? It would seem that those who have the power for our health care delivery systems will bear no responsibility for its outcomes.

Here is where our expectations become a part of the problem. Often I hear folks complain about their practitioners, for example, about laboratory results. You may assume that the doctor's office will call you with your results, but they don't. You then assume that since they didn't call, everything must be all right. A year goes by and at the obligatory office visit, you are informed that you had an abnormal finding on your laboratory results. The faultfinding begins, leading to outrage. But is it realistic to have this expectation? It gets back to that old "assume" rule. In truth, your peace of mind is your responsibility. We cannot assume that our welfare is someone else's priority. It must be our own.

The health insurance industry, with all of its cumbersome rules, has generated less care for more cost. Health care providers embody caring. This is a part of the paradox. One part (doctors and nurses) of the system cares deeply about the patient. The other part (insurance company and the third party payer) cares only about cutting costs. The caregivers, not the care-restrictors, present the public relations face of health care. It is customary for blame to be affixed to the provider for delays in treatment when it should be laid at the feet of the insurance industry. The third-party-payer system is interested in the financial bottom line. Delay, restrictions, and rationing are their tour de force.

Now more than ever we need to come to terms with personal responsibility in the work of creating health. The challenge of creating physical health resides with you. Your actions are your testimony.

## More Puzzles

With all of the myths around nutrition and our own cultural bias, how do we begin processing the changes we need to make? We need to look at all the rules that govern our dietary life. A good way to do this is to begin keeping a diet diary. Before you begin a diet reformation, it is helpful to get a full look at what you are consuming now. Then you might consider the principles that determine why you eat and what you eat. Those ideas reflect a whole body of human experience that is specific to your family and the community to which you belong.  We need to look at all of those parts of the collective belief systems that determine what you do with food and why you continue to do it.  Some of these concepts will lead us into ways of being.  For instance, the idea of not wasting food, saving leftovers, and cleaning your plate are examples of some food rules.  Buying large quantities "on sale," even something you don't need  now, is another form of a food rule.  There are more, to be sure.

The dynamics of human nutrition do not follow these food rules, yet we avoid like the plague learning about these dynamics.  We will rely on the books from the bookstore and not question how these concepts were developed.  Most of the time, these concepts go to the same old tired behaviors of portion control/will power/and exercise.   Fat oxidation does not occur in that concept.  The proof is in our population.

The influence of nutrients on our physiology is the entire issue.  Nutrients set in motion specific physiologic events that determine what will and will not happen with weight management.  This is all tied into insulin and its resistance by your own body as it is now.  This insulin effect will change as you age and as you are exposed to nutrients.  Even as you attain an ideal body size, your insulin response and reaction times will not remain constant.

There is great wisdom in allowing things to happen as they do.  Often I am engaged in conversations about the theory of insulin resistance and how to use it to best health advantage.  I might make some strong declarations about how exercise doesn't work in getting weight loss.  Usually by this time, I am seeing the listener's eyes glaze over.  Hoping to maintain good communication, I suggest that the person continue doing what they are doing and see what happens.  In a few months I am asked to help them understand why they haven't lost weight.  I might ask them for a diet diary, and the eyes glaze over.  More time goes by.  The riddle of the low-fat-high-carbohydrate diet plus exercise has a very predictable punch line.  It is weight gain and sickness.  At some point I will begin to work with someone who is about to give up, yet for one more try.  This is not a big mystery to solve.  It can be felt in the subtle muscular changes as the effects of our nutritional dynamic impact us.  This is an individual story and it is very specific.  The target is insulin resistance.  We need to understand it, and accept it as the compass of our body.  Insulin resistance is both the cause and the cure of the obesity epidemic.

Staying in the puzzle is a form of intellectual resistance.  In other words, we will only allow change to occur in our life at the rate at which we understand "why".  This means time will have to stand still until your questions are resolved.  Then as little bits of acceptance on your part begin to gain hold, slowly you begin.  Even cautious progress will be seasoned with portion control.  I have seen people refuse to look at the scale.  They do not want to know what they weigh.  If you don't acknowledge it, you can't change it.  If you don't accept your weight/wait, you cannot get into taking effective action steps.  There is a Buddhist paradigm about right thought, right vision, right feeling, and right action.  Its message is self-explanatory.

How nice is it to leave behind that old tired victim who demands to know why things happen as they do.  It has been my observation that one can heal without knowing why.  One's sense of faith in a plan bigger than the human mind can create is often forged from the fires of "why."  Learning how to live when life doesn't make sense is our challenge. Holding onto the center when the going is tough defines us. We can always perform well when life is going along in step with our plans. We can even lose weight when we have lots of money in the bank and everybody is healthy. Stress comes in from some source and we cave in. What defines us is how we manage in adversity. We need to rise to the occasion. Reframing adversity can change a negative into a positive. It's how you are willing to look at it.

**Delay is Futile**

The incredible human body has a limitless ability to heal on its own. It does this many times over. We take it for granted until it stops.

Delay, waiting, postponing, self-imposed limitations, and justifications (weight/wait) are ways we use to control the rate at which we will allow change to occur in our life.

Often it is said, "As soon as I get time to figure this out, or take this trip, or have my birthday, or get enough money, then I will work at getting healthy."

The health-related consequences of delay are numerous. We all know of those who waited too long to do something. Getting healthy now becomes a simple matter of making careful, planned choices every day.

Most challenging of all is accepting your part in making choices crucial to your health. They require personal responsibility, ownership, integrity, and creativity. Blaming someone else is a way of dodging your responsibility.

# Why You Can't Have Your Cake & Eat It, Too

Avoiding your health issues or your weight issues is prolonging your recovery. Many of us have a strong will to live. However, we disconnect from the will to heal. This requires work. It is something we must do for ourselves. It is not done to us or for us.

## A New Paradigm

It is vital that you learn what food is. Just like words, food has a definable quality. These qualities are protein, fat, and carbohydrates. This means that each food type will set in motion a very individualized reaction. This personalized reaction is based on your family medical history and where your body has stored its fat reserves. You can't outrun your genes or your insulin resistance.

First one must understand the types of food. Second, to appreciate the densities of these items. There is no mystification needed here. Protein is protein. Fat is fat. Carbohydrates are carbohydrates.

As you begin to learn the values of food in terms of what it is, then it is vital to learn about the differences in the densities of food as expressed in the cooked weights and calories. Food has a direct impact on our physiology. This impact is very different from the slick mystification of the "impact carbohydrate" that we are now seeing in the marketing of low carbohydrate foods. In order to get us to buy products like ice cream and candy bars dressed up like protein bars, we are told the impact carbohydrate value is very low. This value is less than 2 grams of carbohydrate, for example, per serving. We are led to believe that maltitol or sugar alcohols wrap a Teflon-like shield around these sugars so they won't raise blood sugar or blood insulin.  We know from experience and from scientific laboratory testing that this claim is completely false.

So learning the impact of nutrients on cellular functioning opens up the development of the insulin connection to the symptoms we experience. Insulin is the arbiter of weight management.  This is  insulin resistance and glucose toxicity in your body as it manifests today.  This is the core issue in the creation of the human diseases emerging in the acquired maladies of our time.  These maladies include non-insulin-dependent diabetes, sleep apnea, high blood pressure, high triglycerides, high cholesterol, irritable bowel syndrome, headache, cravings, asthma, indigestion, and obesity.

We need to download a new program into the collective mind. For the last five decades the portion-control, calorie-counting, exercise, more will power program has pervaded the entire cultural mind.  It exists in newspapers, magazines, marketplace, families, and business.  This program is found in families, medical schools, and nutritional education. Cultures will have their own mythology.  Television programs replicate this thinking in a myriad of forms.  The higher learning institutions perpetuate this erroneous program.  The institutions that are created to support diabetes, heart disease, and cancer support and are supported by these food theories.

In working with patients, I always ask them why it is they have gained weight.  Without fail they relate that they have been a failure at portion control, will power, and exercise.  Then I ask them to relate what methods they have tried to obtain weight loss.  Most say they already exercise every day and try to eat healthy food.    They may even relate all of the commercial diets they have tried and failed.    At some point they may regard themselves as moral failures because they have been unable to conquer this particular demon.    In a symbolic way, they embody the sense of failure for these erroneous belief systems.

When I share with them the concept of insulin resistance as the prime mover in weight management, they respond with relief.  It all makes sense, they say.  When I relate the truth about the impact of exercise on weight management, some of my patients have wept.  For all of their days as an obese person, they have bought into the exercise-to-lose-weight belief system.  They have only to look at the results of these belief systems to see that for them, they just don't work.

Insulin resistance and glucose toxicity are individual patterns that are reflected in the full spectrum of adult-onset disease and obesity.  Younger populations are afflicted with insulin resistance with alarming frequency.  There are now normal-weighted, insulin-resistant individuals.  The one common denominator in all of these circumstances is insulin resistance. A second common denominator is the erroneous belief systems of portion control, exercise, and more will power as a way to obtain weight management and health. These two idealized mythologies usually exist simultaneously.

Weight management techniques and health management plans are dependent on managing insulin resistance.  This in turn is dependent on reduction of carbohydrate exposure. Appropriate nutritional education, unlike anything we have been taught in the past, will create the balanced diet we have been seeking. This balanced diet must reflect the individual's medical needs, and his ideal body weight.    Unless we are willing to give up the food pyramid, portion control mythology, and exercise as the sole arbiters of weight management and health, we are doomed.  For all the advances in technology, our issues with food will be our demise.

Sometimes I see this culture as hopelessly entrenched in its mythological nutritional, medical, and exercise belief systems. Symbolically, we are seeing groups of animals beaching themselves in a suicidal pact.  I ask myself, are we like these creatures?  Do we continue to follow a belief pattern even though it is killing us?  Our refusal to change these old tapes and our resistance to learning something new is significant. Our mental stubbornness and our physical systems are a reflection of our insulin resistance. This resistance is reflected in physical disease and excess body fat.

Delay is a luxury we cannot afford as a culture if we are to conquer insulin resistance.    Stubbornness will mean a constant steady decline in health and a way of life.  We cannot afford declining health and losing out on enjoying life. Be aware that our nutritional deficiency diseases are expressed today.  They are just as dangerous as the ones we conquered in the 1900's.

**Process the Process**

Attaining your ideal body weight, achieving a state of wellness, and improving the quality of your life will depend on the sensitivity in YOUR body to the insulin glucose relationship.  The presence of blood sugar requires pancreatic insulin.  Insulin is an important hormonal symbol/signal, which tells your body that food is plentiful.  Abundant blood sugar means that stored body fat remains in place.  Body fat is the human body's insurance policy against starvation.  In order to consistently utilize body fat, many nutritional conditions must be met, including adequate protein, water, rest, and minimal carbohydrate exposure.  Remember that body fat contributes to the caloric expense of the body.  Some of the calories utilized will be from food, and the rest will come from the fat reserves.

By using your ample stores of fat as your primary energy source, you can decrease the fat mass and lose weight.  The primary technique for accomplishing this will be dietary.  In many cases where there is extreme fat storage, utilizing exercise is inappropriate.  The additional weight and strain on the bones and joints can be harmful.  Blood pressure can go dangerously high in insulin-resistant individuals, and there may be a risk of dangerous blood pressure elevations, even during walking.  It is important to obtain a stable blood pressure before taking on a vigorous exercise program.  It is also helpful to have lost a fair amount of stored body fat to ensure a stable balance and protect the joints.  Often in individuals the center of gravity is off due to large fat deposits around the middle of the body, the arms, and the legs, making exercise precarious.

Restoring this "balance" to the body in transition needs to be maintained.  We have often heard about balance and health, but I submit, we don't know what they mean. There is no credible definition for "balanced" or "healthy".  They are words that usually mean more nutritional spin.  These concepts are equally applied to exercise.

# Why You Can't Have Your Cake & Eat It, Too

 Coordinating the time to begin exercise as a part of your wellness routine will depend on the recovery your body makes as it goes through fat loss.  It just doesn't make sense to work out with a body that is currently affected with sleep deprivation due to sleep apnea.  This is one time when it is good to wait and go slowly.  We can agree that protecting your heart and spinal column are very important.  Perhaps this is a healthful balanced approach that is required at the time.  It is important to stay flexible as the situation improves.

One of the areas of concern I have among health professionals is the common belief in exercise as a means to lose weight.  When I share with my colleagues my concepts on wellness, they waste no time in telling me how I need to incorporate exercise into my suggestions.

Even in the family member who is afflicted with a weight issue, they will have a close relative who will insist on strenuous activity as a means to get weight loss.   In both camps there is an operating collective belief system in the way to obtain weight loss.   As family members and as health advocates we need to put our egos aside.  We cannot correct insulin resistance with exercise. It is not possible to lose weight with exercise.  To heal the epidemic of obesity we need to teach the truth about carbohydrates and their effect on the physiology of insulin.

In unprecedented numbers societies all over the world are experiencing problems with obesity and insulin resistance. This type of malnutrition is even more deadly than a lack of food.  More people are dying from over-nutrition than under-nutrition.  It is a fact.  Given another look, both states are a serious form of malnutrition.   How can so many become malnourished?  Many theories may be suggested, but there is one common denominator - insulin resistance.  We are creating a state of extreme nutritional disease.  This is just like the days when scurvy and rickets ravaged the malnourished.

The food supply is limitless.  There are many choices available in our markets from all over the world.  The food supply is protected by safe handling techniques that continue to evolve and improve.  Fresh food is still the paradigm of the palate.  Discerning chiefs demand fresh ingredients.  The truth of the matter is that the majority of us rarely eat fresh food.  Most of the food consumed today is consumed in the car or in a restaurant.  We are becoming dependent on processed food while we relinquish our skills as cooks.  With gallows-like humor, we scoff at those who cook their own food and eat at home.

Cooking meals in the home is one skill that has become eroded by the have-it-now fast food culture. We need to remember that obtaining food is something we must do outside the home.  We need transportation to visit the market or to get fast food.  It is an obvious fact, that to eat at a restaurant, one needs to drive and have lots of money.  This type of feeding is very expensive.  There comes a day when infirmities may cause problems with driving.  We are not stable on our feet or able to handle bodily functions in public.  Driving a car, going to the food store, and creating home cooked meals now become important in the quality of life.  However this reality unfolds, we find by our circumstances we cannot support ourselves at home.  Having the ability to cook and obtain fresh ingredients becomes a life saving skill.

# Why You Can't Have Your Cake & Eat It, Too

Our aging populations are becoming desperately malnourished. They are becoming nutritionally deficient and severely dehydrated. While it may not be viewed that way, extreme malnutrition occurs when folks cannot get out to get fresh food. Dehydration follows when folks fear frequent trips to the bathroom. Perhaps it is better said that it is inconvenient to have to use the bathroom. So there are folks who deliberately withhold water. Dehydration brings confusion and depression to its victims. Early low-level dehydration is often dismissed as just getting old. Early low-level malnutrition is often dismissed or missed completely. Our society has "pathologized" and mythologized just about everything. Fresh water and fresh food are important life-enhancing elements. These simple things will improve many cases of human suffering. We believe in pills more than common sense.

It is not unusual to hear about individuals who drink less than 8 ounces of water a day. They have dry wrinkled skin and suffer from constipation. It is not unusual for these folks to be placed on large numbers of prescription drugs including a diuretic. I heard a woman on an elevator deriding her physician's direction to drink at least a quart of water before returning for her next office visit. As she made her comments her friends supported her laughing at the suggestion to drink water.

## Chapter Two:
## Defining The Elements

## Putting The Elements Together

You are embarking on a process that has many elements. These involve careful shopping, preparation, and advance planning. Trying, staying willing, and holding the heart kindly will go far in your personal development. A spirit of enthusiasm will guide you as we measure the progress you make week-by-week, month-by-month. This becomes a journey into attaining an ideal. It happens one day at a time, and is done with great courage. Remember your waiting creates weight.

Create a shopping list and a preparation timetable. There are some suggestions later on in this guide. There is no shortcut way to stock the pantry or refrigerator. Keeping fresh food on hand is as important as keeping reserves. The hurry-up lifestyle has imposed shortened preparation times and mealtimes. Somewhere embedded in our DNA there is a memory of savoring meals and enjoying the camaraderie around the table. This is an important part of nourishing the human spirit. Experience has taught me the impact of this kind of deficiency on the health and wellness of individuals. We talk about vitamin deficiencies and how to remedy them. A validation deficiency is as apparent as any vitamin deficiency. Preparing and sharing a meal is a nourishing activity, just as much as food.

One of the elements worthy of incorporating into your wellness routine is accountability. The issue here is transparency. This means your behavior with food is the same in private as it is in public.

After I describe to you the process of insulin resistance, it then becomes an activity requiring your involvement. Our hurry-up double-time culture has mandated the fast-fix response to our health riddles. This just simply will not work. We also are hooked into instant gratification and reward. Being satisfied is another way we interpret the experience of eating. Bringing healing to our attachments means we are willing to look at satisfaction, reward, and gratification differently.

Each day you will be asked to keep an accounting of how you have made food choices, either on paper or mentally. Two infallible measuring tools will place a value on your weight management techniques and will also tell us how quickly you are changing your belief systems. They are the scale and the tape measure. Weight loss does not occur in a vacuum. Results indicate actions. Accountability is a personal skill. Being accountable is a remedy for procrastination. If we are to obtain corrections to your body size and health issues you will have to be accountable.

Many of the mystical traditions have considered the solar plexus as an important energy center. It is located in the middle of the abdomen and is sometimes referred to as the Third Chakra. The organs found in this energy center are the liver, pancreas, stomach, and spleen, all of primary importance in the activity of nutrition and immunity. We often refer to a knowing in our gut, or a gut-wrenching experience. The symbolic interpretation of the gut experience is inner integrity, and when it speaks to us, we all know we should not ignore its wisdom. This visceral wisdom is trying to tell us something important about regaining our health as people and as a nation.

We can no longer be indiscriminate as we ingest substances and food. We will not be able to afford to save time by eating inappropriate foods at breakneck speed. Time and money are the currency in this relationship. Our indifference to our personal responsibility for our health has a trickle-down effect on the health of our economy. It will exact the price of time from the value of life.

As this large segment of the population afflicted with obesity gets into the disabling effects of insulin resistance, the economy of the family will be impacted. The time and money needed to care for these individuals will strain the resources of the entire community -- the business community, the healthcare community, and the family -- all will bear the workload when 65% of the population is in need of care and out of the productive workforce.

Inner accountability and personal responsibility reside in the solar plexus. It is an amazing coincidence that this is where the major digestive organs reside. Therefore, don't wait too long to get started. You may find slow elimination of problem foods may be an effective way to get started. For some of us, clearing out the pantry of problem foods may seem wasteful. So we continue to use these items until they are gone. While this may make sense in terms of economics, it contradicts the basic quality of personal responsibility. Throwing away food or continuing to use problem foods are not the only alternatives available to you.

# Why You Can't Have Your Cake & Eat It, Too

This is one of our cultural belief systems.  We should not waste food.  Eliminating toxic foods from our immediate environment may seem wasteful.  The big picture, however, is that these foods will sabotage your effort.  Donate them to the food bank in your area and don't replenish the supply.  Don't wait to do this. Procrastination is a form of wait and weight.  It is measured in terms of pounds and inches and time.

## Nutritional Values: Food as Energy

There are only two food groups -- foods with calories and foods without calories.  Of the foods with calories there are three types, namely, protein, carbohydrates, and fat.  Protein has 4 calories per gram.  Carbohydrates have 4 calories per gram, and fat has 9 calories per gram.  There is no differentiation for simple, complex, organic, or "healthy." The words good or bad also are not used.  To date the human body has no computer chips installed to notify it of these marketing buzzwords.  The amazing human body has a way of using nutrients that has to do with their type and not speed of their use.  The stomach does not read labels and is not influenced by any of the clever marketing adjectives used to describe food.  Natural, balanced, or anti-oxidant are terms our biology cannot '"read".  Our bodies are looking for protein, fat, carbohydrates, and water. Take note also that alcohol has 7 calories per gram and is treated as a fat by the body.

Of the nutrients without calories there are two.  One of those nutrients is water.  Water is perhaps the most important of all the nutrients we have.  It cools us, removes waste, supports all the streams of energy from the organ systems, and quenches our thirst. Water is vital to our alertness and our states of wellness.  It is a natural appetite suppressant.

# Why You Can't Have Your Cake & Eat It, Too

The other nutrient includes the vitamins and minerals group. Another way to address this group is to call them micronutrients. It is just not possible to consume recommended daily requirements of micronutrients from food. It could be done, but this task would require us to eat copious amounts of food all day long. This would have obvious consequences. Multivitamins, calcium, salt, and potassium are the important micronutrients that can be obtained in supplement form. A word of caution here is necessary. The supplement industry has become saturated with "snake oil" artists. I have seen very intelligent people pay $130 for a 30-day supply of vitamins when there was a similar product available for $12. Be careful when shopping for these items.

In the hierarchy of usage, nutrients have a very specific order. Carbohydrates must be used first because they require insulin to bind to them. This insulin response cannot be avoided or interrupted by any clever food-combining scheme, nor subjugated by exercise. Think of insulin as a large boom-box with its sound cranked to the highest volume. The vibration and volume are intense. Portion control and calorie-counting have no effect on controlling the level of power from insulin. It is a commanding signal. Abatement of insulin will occur when carbohydrates are restricted. Abatement of insulin resistance will occur when insulin is not needed to manage dietary influxes of carbohydrate. We need to quiet the insulin signal by turning down the volume on carbohydrate intake. This is a very simple way to tell the story of insulin resistance and glucose toxicity. Sometimes using a simple story as a metaphor can bridge the gap in understanding a scientific complexity. This metaphor is a simple way to connect to the mystery of insulin resistance and all of its counterparts.

# Why You Can't Have Your Cake & Eat It, Too

Protein has its place in priority of usage.  The human body needs protein, but It cannot store it.  Therefore, protein must be replaced every day.  While the tempest is taking place, the body will still need protein.  It is at these times that the body may elect to use its own parts for protein.  This drama creates tissue destruction.  The eyes, kidneys, muscles, and even the heart can be targets for this effort.  Remember, your body is trying to keep going.  It will sacrifice itself to do that.

Fat is the body's preferred fuel source, a plentiful energy-rich commodity.  The wonderful human body is hardwired to burn its fat.  Carbohydrates and its cohort insulin corrupt this effort.  The degree of resistance generated by your body is going to determine how deep the corruption of fat oxidation will be.  In other words, insulin prohibits the body from burning fat.  The absence of insulin or limiting it will enhance fat oxidation.  This is metabolism doing its thing.  It needs our cooperation.

## The Case for Water

Water is vital to the body.  Plasma, cerebrospinal fluids, perspiration, and many more vital body fluids are made of water.  The fluid dynamic of the body to cool itself, rid itself of waste, and carry nutrients all require water.    It is suggested to drink 3 quarts, 96 ounces, 12 8-ounce glasses of water per day. Begin by drinking amounts of water that are comfortable for you.  Some of us can drink water by the quart at a sitting.  Others drink it in small amounts.  Listen to your subtle thirst detector, and know your limits.  Learning when you are thirsty, and when you are well hydrated will be a part of this journey.  Try to drink all of your water before 6 p.m., or at least four hours before you retire for the night.    Getting a good night's rest is very important.    The consequence of going to the bathroom all night needs to be avoided. If your water intake is not completed before 6 or 7 p.m., then just stop. Start over the next day.

Water promotes functioning of the liver, plumps the skin, and helps to remove waste. Thirst is a motivator for the stimulus of hunger. Many of us learn we were eating (salty or sweet) when we were thirsty. Dehydration is a chronic problem for those who are living in arid climates and climate-controlled areas. Difficulty with energy levels, headache, and constipation are related to how we maintain our water reserves. Sustaining fat loss is dependent on the intake of water. The liver requires large amounts of water to do the work of fat oxidation. Keeping a constant supply of water in you is a way to manage hunger triggers, and to keep us hydrated in the extremes of temperature our climates.

Many of us are chronically dehydrated and don't know it. We ride in air-conditioned vehicles, whether cars or airplanes, and work in air-conditioned buildings. These environments dehydrate us. High altitudes create intense evaporation in the body. In some ways these types of environments are like deserts. While we think we are cool, we are really losing lots of water. People who work outside continually drink water. For those of us who work inside, we usually drink soft drinks or coffee, further dehydrating us. This is a serious health problem.

We all understand how individuals become dehydrated out in the harsh southwest deserts. They go through various stages before they succumb. They may become cold, confused, depressed, before they collapse. We are seeing these symptoms of confusion and depression in the clinical setting.

# Why You Can't Have Your Cake & Eat It, Too

The symptoms may be and indication of dehydration, rather than something pathological.  Constipation is also an issue with dehydration.  Again and again, these symptoms are medicated before they are investigated.  It doesn't make sense to give diuretics and laxatives to folks that are not drinking enough water.  But, it happens all the time.

Write down how much water you drink each day as pure water.  This is an important way to discover how you are managing the intake of water.  Carbonated beverages, coffee, tea, and alcoholic beverages are not water.  These things do not hydrate, but act to further dehydrate the body.

It is time to drink your water.  Don't wait.  It is weight.

## Vitamins and Minerals

The other nutrients without calories are vitamins and minerals, which are vital to the maintenance of intrinsic cellular functioning. They are impossible to ingest in therapeutic levels from the food we eat. For instance, ten oranges would yield 1000 mg of Vitamin C, which would be a significant source of carbohydrates in the diet.  Obtaining nutrients from the diet becomes a high-volume-intake proposition.  It is therefore important to include a multivitamin as a part of your daily intake and avoid the increased caloric intake expense. Any multivitamin is fine.

Often this is a place where the discussion turns to the organic versus synthetic debate, which can take many forms. Hydrochloric acid located in the stomach doesn't really care if an item is natural or synthetic.  It will break things down very efficiently and without regard to how much something costs, without the benefit of a computer chip or a scanner. The stomach has been given many mystical qualities. It is a very amazing organ, but it is not the spectrometer of the body. The stomach has not been given glasses so it cannot read all the publicity that flows on the media. The stomach does not have a turnstile in it to direct things into a good and bad place in the system. It just doesn't work that way.

Try to avoid getting sucked into paying a fortune for these supplements. The supplement industry has profited from our gullibility. They make up all kinds of mythology to create fear and insecurity in us. What we need to know is that the food supply is not going to supply us with the micronutrients we need. It would be nice if this was true, but it is not.

## Calcium Replacement

Calcium is very important. We are going to need it in amounts the diet is just not able to provide. Use elemental calcium supplements such as Caltrate-D, Citri-cal, or some other over-the-counter types of calcium. Look for a calcium citrate with magnesium and vitamin D. These things are easily absorbed and work well in the prevention of bone loss. Avoid calcium that is made from oyster shells or coral, as these forms of calcium are indigestible. It is basically like swallowing rocks or chalk. We would not intentionally swallow a shell or a piece of coral.

Milk does supply calcium but not enough to be considered therapeutic. An 8-ounce glass of milk will provide about 100 mg of calcium. It will also contain 12 grams of lactose or sugar. Milk is available in many strengths of fat content. Whether the milk is full fatted or skim, does not change its lactose content. The lactose content will stimulate insulin just like white sugar in the bowl. Our altered perceptions about wholesomeness apply to the entire dairy category. It is almost sacred. In many ways it is like the "sacred cow" of nutrition. Yogurt and milk are the sacred cows of the diet. The truth of the matter with these items is that they contain a lot of sugar. Oh, sure, we say, this is "natural" or wholesome. We have a huge advertising campaign centered on milk and how it is a valuable asset to a weight-loss plan. We need to remember that milk is mostly sugar. It will act like sugar creating problems with its uptake and the disposal of insulin. This will retard fat use and create a host of metabolic disturbances in susceptible individuals.

Take at least 1200 mg of calcium per day. Remember that calcium interferes with the absorption rates for anything that is in the stomach. It should be taken alone with food and lots of water. Be aware of this when taking your prescription drugs.

## Potassium Replacement

One other very important mineral is potassium. This element is a part of the chemical message system that innervates the muscles. When potassium levels are decreasing the following symptoms appear: feeling tired, feeling cold, muscle cramps in the large muscles of the body, and constipation. The high-protein low-carbohydrate eating plans eliminate a lot of the foods that would be higher in potassium. The banana and the potato represent a contribution of 600 mg of potassium depending on the size. These items will also contribute a significant amount of sugar into the diet. This will create the insulin response that we know will interfere with fat oxidation. It may also severely elevate blood sugar in diabetics.

# Why You Can't Have Your Cake & Eat It, Too

The symptoms of potassium depletion may be experienced as muscles cramp in the hands, or the lower legs. Feeling cold, abdominal distention, and headache may also indicate that the body is getting low in potassium. The RDA's for potassium are 3600 mg. This means one would have to eat six bananas or potatoes. If we were trying to get potassium from spinach we would need to eat five cups of cooked spinach.

I wish it were as simple as getting prescription strength potassium to assist in the replacement of potassium. There are many conditions that must be met before the physician will order potassium replacements. Most of the time, the belief is that potassium should be replaced by food. This would be inappropriate for those who are trying to manage their weight and their blood sugars. Blood values need to be checked as well to ascertain what the status of potassium is at the time. This is a way to measure where the blood potassium is before and during the treatment. There is a potassium phobia in the medical community. There are instances of restless leg syndrome being treated with strong anti-psychotic drugs when simple potassium replacement is all that is required. This is also true of many of the "neuropathies" that are becoming popular today.

Please do not underestimate the vital importance of serum potassium. Potassium depletions can result in heartbeat irregularities, which can be serious. There are instances of irregular heartbeats with low normal serum potassium levels. Fluctuations to the serum potassium levels will typically create exhaustion, feelings of being cold, and headache before they get more progressive. Be aware of these subtleties.

# Why You Can't Have Your Cake & Eat It, Too

There are some very good over-the-counter potassium supplements.   Health food store potassium is supplied in 90 mg tablets as potassium chloride.   The regulations on OTC potassium are such that only the smallest doses can be sold. The prescription strength potassium supplement is provided in 750 mg to 1500 mg doses.   In order to obtain adequate potassium replacement from the OTC types, just do the math.

Emergence is another product available containing 200 mg of potassium per dose.   It comes as a powder to be dissolved in water.  This makes it another way to get all of the water in as well.  After the powder is dissolved in water you will find that it fizzes.   There is only one sugarless type of Emergence, so that one would be suitable for the low carb diet.  It is quite refreshing in the lemon-lime flavor.   For severe restless legs or leg cramps try using more than one packet of the Emergence at a time.

Lately protein drinks are being made with significant amounts of potassium added to them.  Be sure to check the product label to see if the protein replacement drink you are using has enough potassium.  Using the protein drinks for  nutrition and potassium supplementation makes them especially beneficial.

## Regulating Regularity

The primary source of your energy intake will be in the form of protein.  The common mythology is that the protein style of dieting will produce constipation.  We have been led to believe that fiber from grain products, such as cereal, is the panacea for constipation. There are several realities here that need to be addressed. Protein-rich diets are not the cause of constipation.   Constipation is the result of inadequate water and oil in the diet.   Oil and water, two important elements to hydrate and lubricate the bowel are all that is needed to get bowel function restored.  Walking also helps.

There are some good psyllium-type fiber bowel bulking laxatives.  Fibercon is very safe and can be taken frequently during the day to keep the bowel active.  Most of us have been dehydrated and become fat-phobic.  These two issues are basic with restoring bowel function.   If you have a trusted remedy, keep it handy.  It is good to keep your bowel function at an optimal state.  We need to be careful in maintaining a regular time and allowing enough time to take care of this important function.  Many of us are in too big a hurry to spend the time we need to in the bathroom.

The low-fat high-carbohydrate pyramid scheme has resulted in chronic bowel discomfort for many of us.  It has been either constipation or diarrhea with lots of distention in between.  This has been called Irritable Bowel Syndrome, which is nothing more than the product of the high-carbohydrate eating style.

There are various types of bowel care preparations.  Some laxatives will pull large amounts of water out of the body to add water to the stool.  This sometimes produces a large result and expels a lot of water.  Sometimes folks believe that they have lost a lot of weight when really they have simply lost water.   This water loss is quickly regained when water is added into the diet.  One example of this is Milk of Magnesia.  Other laxatives add fiber to the stool so that it bulks up.  This will generate a bowel movement due to the increase in size of the stool mass. Some of those types are Fibercon, Metamucil,

# Why You Can't Have Your Cake & Eat It, Too

Citrucel, and Perdiem.  Most of these fiber-type bowel preps are available as sugar free.  Remember to get sugar free items as much as possible.

Lastly, there are irritant-type laxatives. These will stimulate peristalsis, meaning they will act like a cattle prod to the bowel.  For sluggish bowel function this can be helpful, but one will need to be very careful to avoid cramping and pain. The idea here is to obtain as normal a movement as possible.

Be sure to read the directions on over-the-counter bowel care products.   Metamucil, Citrucel, Fibercon, and Perdiem may be taken up to four times a day.  The irritant-type laxatives should be taken with much more caution.  One important feature is to avoid using the irritant-type laxative regularly. For some of us it is necessary to allow the appropriate amount of time to have a bowel movement.  Sometimes we are in a hurry, under stress, or behind schedule.  Plan your daily routine to take care of business in the bathroom.  Be sure to drink lots of water and add fat to your diet if you are troubled with constipation.

One of the most troubling side effects of the high-carbohydrate low-fat eating plan, is irritable bowel syndrome. This syndrome will appear as either loose frequent stools, or constipation.  As soon as you are able to correct this high carbohydrate eating, you will see an appreciable difference in the way the bowel is functioning.  Most of the time, you will experience a restoration to near normal bowel functioning. Remember this key point, water and oil are the most important elements in eliminating waste from the body.

# Why You Can't Have Your Cake & Eat It, Too

## Food Familiarity:  Read labels

Locate and familiarize yourself with the values in the foods you are now eating, as well as the foods you will be eating. There are some good references at your local bookstore in the nutrition section.  These references will also have listings for meals found in local restaurants and fast-food places. Look for references that contain listings of the grams of protein, carbohydrates, and fat in the item, as well as the caloric values.  Much as we have dictionaries to teach us the meaning of words, food has a specific meaning to our body.

Quite simply, we have misperceived food.  The misperceptions about food go the type of food, how it is used, and the amounts of caloric value.  As we investigate these food values, it is important to have a clear understanding of its primary make-up.  For instance, peanut butter is the most misperceived food.  Most folks think of it as a protein.  If one looks up its values you will see that it is primarily made of fat containing equal small amounts of protein and carbohydrate. The nut category will reveal a similar pattern in all nuts.  If we are looking for a fatty food with carbohydrates and protein, then nuts would be suitable.  Nuts contain some protein it is true, but when we are attempting a serious improvement in overall protein intake, nuts supply a minimal amount.

As you become acquainted with these values, the impact of your choices both past and present become very important.  It is like an archeological dig into your nutrition.  It is a way to solve our health mysteries, and assist us in learning the meaning of food.  Avoiding this step is very costly to the process of getting healthy. We have to get the blinders off

# Why You Can't Have Your Cake & Eat It, Too

when it comes to food values, and food categories.  Food needs to be de-mystified so you can get quickly  to the bottom line in the effect of that food on your particular physiology. Mystifications of food appear in the form of adjectives like organic, whole, natural, healthy, time-release, impact, good, or bad.   These words are meaningless when it comes to the digestion if food.

You should look for a book of nutrition facts that will act like a huge database for you.  We are going to need to know food composition without any bells and whistles.   Corrine Netter is an author who provides a Complete Book of Food Counts. Nutribase also is an excellent source for food compositions. Nutribase Nutrition Facts also has an online resource but it is very expensive to download and maintain.   The hand-held computers are beginning to develop programs for keeping track of dietary intake.  Often these programs will provide food compositions in grams and calories.   This foundation will be important as you gain an understanding of food and its functioning in your body today.

One of the common misperceptions about beans, rice, and milk is that these foods supply protein.   Yogurt is also commonly believed to be a protein source.  While these foods do have a small amount of protein content, they are 75% carbohydrate. These carbohydrate-rich foods become sugar in very fast order. Because they have the surreal aura of health around them, they become a sacred staple of the diet. This sacred aura is also around cereal, one of the most commonly misinterpreted types of food.  This is probably due to the extensive advertising of this product.   Cereal costs hardly anything to make, but costs a fortune to buy.  The most valuable thing about cereal is the box.    Make no mistake;

cereal in all forms is sugar. Think of it as a box of miniature donuts. Even with milk on it, it is mostly sugar. If you add fruit to it, is has more sugar. Oatmeal, the holy grail of the so-called healthy diet, is hot sugar.

Keeping records is one of the most important aspects of the archeology of your diet. The past nutritional habits need to be evaluated for you to understand how you evolved physically. This will also aquatint you with food values. As you begin your recovery diet, it will be vital to diagram your food intake. This will act like a mirror reflecting food values onto your results. Many times writing down the food intake will astonish and surprise you. Many people are astonished when they learn on their own how little water and protein they are consuming. Many people are shocked when they discover how much carbohydrate they are ingesting daily. Keeping a food diary from the beginning of this work will help you learn how to integrate a recovery food plan into your diet. It is a way to make certain you are meeting your minimal protein needs, your maximal carbohydrate needs, your maximal fat needs, plus water, and vitamins. Getting the required water, vitamins, and protein will be the vital key to attaining ideal body weight and optimal health.

Sometimes the act of picking up the pen will cut short the out-of-control and stress-related eating patterns. All of us can make excuses, justify, and delay just about anything. But once the pen hits the paper and the calculations are made, denial of the evidence is impossible.

# Why You Can't Have Your Cake & Eat It, Too

Here are some diet bytes:

- Before you bite it- write it!!!

- If it is white, don't bite it!!!

- If you don't know what it is, don't bite it!!

- If you don't want to know what it is, don't bite it!!!

- If it is a mystery food, don't bite it.

- Fat Free means high sugar, high carbohydrate, and low protein content!

- When in doubt, don't bite it!

## Reviewing Labels

Looking at labels and evaluating them will reveal to you some very carefully crafted fictional labeling which takes place on food labels today. Recently there has been a proliferation of a few new fabrications, such as something called "non-impact carbohydrates."  Other new descriptions are "sugar alcohol," maltitol, and glycerin.  These items appear with a certain level of reassurance and authority. The claim that they do not raise blood sugar is completely false.  We know unequivocally that these foods will raise blood sugar.  (Remember, blood sugar stimulates insulin release.)  In practice these ingredients, including fiber, do raise blood sugar and also have a definite caloric value.

There is a low-carb beer on the market now.  It makes the claim of containing 2.9 grams of carbohydrate, yet the label states there is a total of 96 calories in an 12-ounce serving. The bottle holds twelve ounces. Does anyone drink one beer? Rounding out the total stated grams of carbohydrate to 3 grams and multiplying by 4 for the number of calories per gram, we get a total of 12 calories. Subtract the 12 from 96 and the remainder is 84 calories. The beer has 84 calories of something that is not defined nor counted. It cannot be pure alcohol, so what is it? Oil? Beef? I will let you make your own assessment of this kind of fabrication and its effect on someone's blood sugar or other blood values. The total carbs in low carb beer is 26 grams per 12 ounces. It is a better choice than the full carb beer but it would be nice if they told the truth in the first place.

This same fuzzy math is seen on the accounting for protein bars. The ingredient glycerin is shown plainly on the label to contain 4.32 calories but is claimed as a non-impact calorie. Hmm. The total number of calories for the glycerin and the maltitol is left off of the label. The total calories will reflect it, however. Confused yet? That is what it is all about. If you can be kept confused for a little while, you might try the product. Protein bars in general are candy bars. The energy carbohydrate bars, energy bars, are all sugar and need to be treated just like candy.

Many of my diabetic patients will go to the health food store looking for a protein staple. The clerk will assure them that the protein bars will not raise blood sugar. Soon the patient is walking out of the store with a case of these bars, which they begin to use liberally. It doesn't take too long for them to see the change in the blood sugars, and their weight gain. One of my patients had an 18-pound weight increase with an increase in her A1c after four months of protein bars. She neglected to relate the fact that she had been consuming two protein bars a day for some time.  She believed what she was told by the store clerk.

One day I was in a so-called health food store where a customer was asking for some supplements that indicated he had joint pain.  The clerk began suggesting all kinds of supplements to the customer, and it sounded very much like dispensing medical advice.  I just couldn't remain silent.

With as much diplomacy as I could gather, I asked the clerk where she had gone to medical school.  She said she had not gone to medical school.  I asked her where she had been to nutrition, nursing, or any related medical training.  She said, she had no such training.  Her education, she said, was in business and the store sent her to a 3-week class on nutrition.

We need to do the work of learning about food.  We cannot assume the clerks in stores or the labels on products are giving us the truth about food.

## Getting On Track

- Weighing and measuring your foods in the beginning is very important to developing an "eye" for the amounts and types of foods you are consuming.  This is also helpful for times when you go out for meals.   When weighing or measuring an item, do so after it is cooked and or drained.

- DO NOT SKIP MEALS.   Always have a back-up plan in the form of a protein drink, or jerky.   Know where some fast food protein choices may be obtained.   Always carry water.

- Preferred methods of preparing foods would be to cook without adding fat or sugar to the recipe.  Broil, steam, or poaching are preferred methods of cooking.

-  Use regular salad dressings, lemon juice, butter, and bouillon. Be sure to avoid dressings and sauces with a lot of carbohydrates and sugar. This means items that contain honey, raspberry syrup, sugar, and corn syrups.  Salsa is a good choice for seasoning.

- Delete from your pantry, shelf, stockpile, and refrigerator all problem foods.  Some of the stuff that probably needs to go is the ketchup, barbeque sauce, butter, crackers, chips and gravies.  Get rid of the cereal, canned soups, and sweets.

- Salad dressings can be purchased from your local grocer. Don't get anything fancy, just get regular dressings or use mayonnaise.  Bleu cheese, ranch dressing, and Caesar are just about the best.  Oil and vinegar always is a good choice.

- Remember barbeque sauce, ketchup, and cocktail sauces are loaded with sugar.

-  Try to remember that low fat means high carbohydrate.

- Try to eat slowly.  Never eat in your car, in front of the TV, while reading, or while at your desk.   We are trying to acquaint you with your stomach, eyes, and your appetite. They need to have your full attention while you are eating.

# Why You Can't Have Your Cake & Eat It, Too

- Be very careful in restaurants.  Ask for broiled foods, prepared without sauces.  Ask that no bread be brought to the table.  And don't forget, salad dressing on the side.

-  Dessert?  Fresh fruit is a good choice.  Work it into your meal plan ahead of time.

- Coffee, tea, and diet soft drinks are fine, used in moderation.  They cannot be counted as water.  Other items that may be included with your water intake are Crystal Lite, herbal tea, sparkling water, bouillon, and sugar-free flavored waters.

- Read labels religiously.  See if the math on the calorie counts adds up.

- Eat when you are not hungry.  This is a way to have good control.  It is something we never do because our cultural bias is to wait until we are hungry before we eat.

Remember, what you eat in private, shows up in public.

## Chapter Three:
## Adding It All Up

## The Importance of Protein

Protein provides the energy that gives your body the fuel it needs while you are oxidizing your fat reserves. Protein intake is calculated in grams and is based on the daily minimum needed amount, as derived from human trials, not from tests on rats. In order to calculate the amount of protein one needs to consume, you must first decide on your ideal body weight. From that, the following equation is developed: IBW (ideal body weight) in Kilograms X 1.5 Gms of protein = the minimal amount of protein in grams to be consumed on a daily basis. Another way to view this amount is to use one gram of protein to one pound of ideal body weight.

The human body does not store protein. It is a fuel-type, which needs to be supplied every day. It is energy, giving you power; it facilitates feeling full and content. All types of protein will be considered in the discussions we will have. Remember that each protein is different in terms of its gram weight. Beef weighs more than shrimp, and so on, meaning the quantities will vary.

Supplying the human body with protein is vital in maintaining energy levels. Protein intake is vital in production of amino acids. Scientists who have studied human nutrition have concluded that a minimal amount of protein must be ingested every day, because it cannot be stored. The formulas will vary, but most practitioners agree on the amounts. This minimal amount of protein is an insurance policy in providing consistent non-insulin-stimulating energy. Protein activates satiation triggers in the gastro-intestinal tract that transmits that "feeling full" idea to the brain.

The protein-modified fast is a strategy recommended for a variety of reasons. It represents a simple but effective feeding technique for significant fat oxidation. Twenty grams of protein 5 to 9 times a day will jump-start a stalled-out weight/wait loss. Simply eat two or three ounces of some kind of protein every two hours. This is to blot out hunger, and keep you regulated. If you are eating every two hours, or three times a day, be sure to get all your protein in every day.

Protein-only dieting can be instituted during busy chaotic times. When choice is crucial, and there isn't a lot to choose from, plan to keep "baggies" of deli style protein slices ready. They can be pre-packed or sliced to order. Liquid proteins may also be used in this way as an effective way to low carb diet, and to improve energy levels. The fast food industry has begun to offer protein burgers and other protein-only fast food items. If fast food is something that you have used in the past, using now may be helpful. By using online food guides you can get information on these food compositions.

There are lots of good reasons to increase your protein intake. You will boost your immune system, decrease your blood sugar, decrease your blood insulin, and improve your fatty acid release. What this does is improve your fat oxidation, and contribute your fat resources to your daily energy output. In other words, you are using your stored body fat for fuel.

One of the signs of protein deficiency is hair loss. Many cases of balding can be traced to a carbohydrate-rich diet.

# Why You Can't Have Your Cake & Eat It, Too

Thinning hair, hair breakage, and other types of hair loss can be a result of lack of protein in the diet. Thinning, brittle, and cracking nails may be the result of low protein intake.  Once we begin increasing the intake of dietary protein, it will take a couple of months to see these areas regroup.

When we are not eating enough protein, we are always hungry. We will have cravings for candy, and starchy foods to take the place of protein.  It doesn't make sense to eat a sleeve of cookies when we want to eat hamburgers. But this is what we do. We have become so protein-phobic that we avoid protein, but we find we are still hungry.  For some reason, we turn to candy, cookies, and chips as a substitute for protein.

 The protein phobias have gathered a lot of energy since the development of the protein-dominated diets.  In the avoidance of protein, we may practice portion control.  There is so much fear about kidney damage from dietary protein, which is completely untrue.  I see many people ration protein out of the mythological fears that dietary protein is destructive to the human body.  Liberal amounts of protein are not toxic to the healthy human body.  Even those having some kidney damage prior to a protein-rich diet, will see improvements in the kidney functions as they make progress.

Protein can be consumed in plentiful amounts.  The carbohydrates need to be controlled.  The intake of carbohydrates will cause huge variations in blood sugar. When the sugar levels in the blood are up, we are "up." When the blood sugar levels in the blood are down, we are downright hungry.  Blood sugar creates a large molecule that has to penetrate the filter of the kidneys.  Because this filter has a very fine screen, blood sugar causes a lot of destruction to the kidney while it is present.

It is an established scientific fact that protein cannot be stored or converted into sugar. Dietary protein is not excreted from the kidneys. Kidney destruction occurs when the body begins to cannibalize itself due to profound high blood sugar and the resultant insulin reaction. The cellular destruction caused by this toxic reaction is well documented in the scientific literature. Protein detected in the urine indicates this fact. This is where the protein phobia got its start.

The dietary history of individuals who consume the typical low-fat high-carbohydrate diet includes very little protein. Typically it would consist of about 500 grams of carbohydrate, 20 grams of protein, and 100 grams or more of fat. People who follow this diet will exhibit, in later stages, varying degrees of disorders such as obesity, non-Insulin-dependent diabetes mellitus, hypertension, and so on.

Just for fun, write down the amount of protein you eat every day. Use the chart on protein to help you determine its weight. Refer to the food composition lists located in the appendix.

## Protein Assessment

| Type | How Much | How Often |
|---|---|---|
| Beef | | |
| Chicken | | |
| Turkey | | |
| Cheese | | |
| Fish | | |
| Cottage cheese | | |
| Protein Drinks | | |
| Eggs | | |
| Totals | | |

# Why You Can't Have Your Cake & Eat It, Too

## The Importance of Carbohydrates

Carbohydrates are always used first by the body for energy because of their insulin-stimulating properties. They are a fuel-type that requires the hormone insulin to bind to it. It is the insulin level that will determine how quickly or how slowly you will progress in the resolution of the disorders you are now facing. When sugar is present, it will interfere with the utilization of fat from the body. By eliminating dietary carbohydrates, you are eliminating most of the sugar from your diet. This will enable your body to burn its fat reserves.

The more carbohydrates you eat, the more sugar stress is applied to the physiological body. This will create pancreatic insulin, and it is the insulin that will stall out fat oxidation by the body. The most toxic substance to the human body is dietary sugar in all forms. The human body tightly regulates its usage. The adult- onset diseases we have are caused by the degrees of blood sugar present and the internal resistance created by the insulin response. The fewer the carbs, the easier it is for your body to function as a fat-burning furnace. Blood sugar gets in the way of fat oxidation. It behaves like an impatient person pushing to get the first place in line.

In the beginning of this plan a 2:1 ratio of protein grams to carbohydrate grams is a good way to find a tolerance level. That means, if you are scheduled to use 120 Gms of protein then you may be able to tolerate 60 grams of carbohydrates. "Tolerate" means your symptoms start to lessen and the weight begins to change. Usually when there is long-standing disease, tolerance of carbohydrates is lessened. Remember, we are committing to a process. We will learn together what YOUR body can tolerate.

# Why You Can't Have Your Cake & Eat It, Too

Under normal conditions, carbohydrates are stored in very limited quantities.  They will be reserved as glycogen (done by the liver) and stored for emergency energy.  The amount of glycogen stored is 3 to 6 pounds depending on the body size.  Glycogen is stored in the blood, muscles and liver.  The only circumstance under which carbohydrates are converted to fat is when fat intake falls below 10 grams per day. It is at this point the body will begin to reserve carbohydrates for fat storage.

Fat is the physical body's insurance policy against starvation.  Fat storage will continue while the body gives up fat during weight reduction.  It is possible to utilize much more fat, when the carbohydrate intake is low provided the amount of dietary fat consumed is kept constant.

This eye-opening experience continues as you go through your first month of high-protein-low-carbohydrate eating.  Patients frequently report the experience of feeling tired, weak, or having low energy.  In the previous eating style (high carbohydrate) you ate frequently and consumed unrestricted amounts of this type of fuel.  Your metabolism was always being charged.  If you had some low energy, typically you would eat more crackers, drink juice, et cetera.  Without the constant carbohydrate replacement, you quite naturally become tired.

How long does it take you to get hungry or tired after your high carbohydrate breakfast?  Most people will relate how hungry they become after the typical banana, bagel, and cereal type breakfast.  They will also report how quickly this hunger and fatigue progresses.   One year this breakfast might last for about 2 hours. The next year it provides sustenance for one hour. The snacking begins as we have this embedded belief that we must wait (there it is again) until lunchtime to eat.

Once you begin to consume much more protein than you now use, you are going to be programmed into your fat reserves. One pound of body fat will provide you with 3500 calories worth of fuel. This is high quality energy. It is like your battery pack is being switched to internal power from an auxiliary power source. The electrical rhythm of your life is returning to its source. You are learning your biorhythms.

Carbohydrate mythologists have told us we need to have sugar for the brain. Did you know that the brain uses 5 mg of glucose an hour? So for 24 hours, the brain uses 120 mg of sugar. A baby aspirin is 81 mg, so you can get a visual of how little sugar an hour the brain actually needs. Another mythology about carbohydrates is the fiber mythology. This particular mythology came about because of problems with constipation or other bowel irregularities. The key point to remember is that our intestinal difficulties are about a lack of water and fat in the diet.

Here is a good place for you to evaluate exactly how much carbohydrate you are now typically eating. Include the variances for weekend eating. Refer to the food composition lists in the appendix.

Remember if it is fat-free, it doesn't contain fat. Most assuredly, it doesn't contain protein. Fat-free foods are always carbohydrates.

# Why You Can't Have Your Cake & Eat It, Too

**Carbohydrate Assessment**

| Type | How Much | How Often |
|---|---|---|
| Fruit | | |
| Pasta | | |
| Bread | | |
| Crackers | | |
| Cereal | | |
| Vegetables | | |
| Beans/Legumes | | |
| Anything Else? | | |
| Totals | | |

# Why You Can't Have Your Cake & Eat It, Too

## Fat Intake while on Plan

The basic formula will allow for a 1:1 ratio of your carbohydrates to your fats. Therefore if your carbohydrate intake is set at 50 Gms, then your fat intake is 50 Gms. Try to go no higher than 60 Gms of fat per day. Fat has the function of keeping food in the gut longer. This gives us the staying power we need to feel "full". The fat discussed here is the added dietary fat. This is the stuff of butter, oils, and grease used for frying. The naturally occurring fat in meats, vegetables, and fruit is not the fat we are measuring. Dairy fat in cottage cheese, or the fat in peanut butter can be helpful. Fat on its own merit, as with protein, does not raise blood sugar.

Dietary fat is always stored. There is no way to pre-empt fat from being stored. Fat is fat. There is no special scanning device anywhere in the human body that differentiates a "good fat" from a "bad fat". If we have created the appropriate eating style for the physiology we have, then it will be possible to burn more fat than can be stored from the diet.

Even the food pyramidists have allowed for ample amounts of fat in the diet. There have been some interesting studies done by researchers looking at the response of the body to fat. Pure fat in the form of oil will not cause blood insulin levels to rise. As with protein, fat does not generate an insulin response. Fat is needed in the diet to prevent the conversions of dietary carbohydrates into triglycerides.

Remember, protein from all sources is about one third fat. Those values are deliberately left off the composition pages.

# Why You Can't Have Your Cake & Eat It, Too

In a subtle way, reversing the "fat free" mentality means consuming large amounts of protein.

Take a moment to evaluate how much fat you are consuming on a daily basis.  Refer to the fat tables in this manual.  Food composition lists are found in the appendix.

**Fat Assessment**

| Type | How Much? | How Often? |
|---|---|---|
| Oils | | |
| Butter | | |
| Fat | | |
| Salad Dressings | | |
| Mayonnaises | | |
| Totals | | |

# Why You Can't Have Your Cake & Eat It, Too

## Getting to Normal

Often the concept "normal" is suggested as some kind of optimal physiologic function with nutrition.  Physiologic function is a fluid process.  It is ongoing and changing daily.  With children, we experience these changes as growth.  With adults, we have the perception that growth has stopped.  This is not the case, for we change in many ways every day.  One of the things heard with loud lament is, "I always could eat thus and so, and it never bothered me before, so how could it be a problem now?"  This is a very unfortunate debate.  It is recycling a belief based on the idea that nothing changes.  We will suspend our efforts to make progress until we have the awareness that a change has indeed occurred.  A lot of us will be unable to move forward at all, until the mysterious change is understood with perfect clarity.   This is the wait in weight.

Well, everything changes.  Even as we look at something, it changes.  Heisinberg introduced us to the principle of uncertainty, which basically says that our perception of a person, place or thing changes it.   Just by looking at something, we change it.   So it is.  With this deep respect for change, it is important to be willing to remain open to discovery.  Keep an open mind as you learn about the subtle changes taking place in your body each and every day.  Your tolerance to carbohydrates in weight maintenance will decrease with time and with your exposure to them.  Your ability to be flexible with your diet and exercise routines will become very important.   These ongoing evaluations are necessary to keep pace with the physiologic changes in your particular situation.  It is a fluid dynamic.

# Why You Can't Have Your Cake & Eat It, Too

Many symptoms and cravings may be alleviated with the initial dietary modifications we have made. Then, one day they may return. This will mean some new sensitivity or intolerance to carbohydrates has developed. It is good to notice how sensitive you have become. Some people describe feeling toxic when eating too many carbohydrates or when the recommended level of carbohydrate exceeds what you can now tolerate. Adjustments to your carbohydrate intake will be the first modification. Always keep your protein intake at your minimal levels, increasing it as needed. Fat intake should remain constant.

With exercise, there can be muscle fatigue. Sometimes sore joints create some problems. The "no pain, no gain" mentality is responsible for much unnecessary suffering. Pain, stiffness, and soreness require attention. These symptoms may necessitate rest or a visit to the medical professional. Remember, it is impossible to lose fat from exercise. It takes 30 miles of walking or running in one day to oxidize one pound of fat.

Exercising to lose weight is another erroneous belief system. It has its roots in our working hard to reach a goal, and is also related to a limiting belief that says to be worthy you must work hard. This "working to be worthy" feeds a lowered sense of self-esteem. Remember, these old belief systems are deeply entrenched in our cultural mind. Just when and where they were introduced into our thoughts is hard to pinpoint. Unfortunately and fortunately, self-esteem is an inside job. What is on the inside shows up on the outside. How we care about ourselves is projected in our demeanor, dress, and disease. The "working hard to be worthy" mentality relates to our dependency on others to give approval for the work you do.   In a very subtle way, others then control the pace at which you will allow yourself to feel good about you.   It is another form of wait/weight.   These errant belief systems, or rules of others, become the collective mind and will control the speed of your getting healthy if you let them. Waiting for approval, is weight.

Old belief systems are like old computer programs.  When we first got computers in our homes and offices, they ran on an operating system we called "DOS".  The maximum memory of these first computers was 40 megabytes.  Today, all of this has changed.  Even as these words are being written, the XP version of Windows will soon be outdated.  The old belief systems are being rewritten.  The old programs we run in our heads are DOS.   We just are getting new "downloads." Portion control, calorie counting, the food pyramid, the glycemic index, exercise to lose weight, food combining, healthy carbs, and getting a balanced diet (whatever that means) are examples of the old programs.  Moreover, they just don't work.

Many times I see the defeated eyes of those who have tried and failed at these old programs.  They embody the failure of these errant belief systems.   I see in the way they carry themselves that they have become the failure themselves. So I just try to get them to remember that these old belief systems are like old computer programs and old computer hardware.  We have new equipment, and we have to use a new program.   We will also have to update these programs when we get new feedback.

Expectations are another form of weight/wait we carry. Remember, expectations generate resentments.   In many ways they can be premeditated, planned, and carried out, leading to disappointment. We will wait or weight for resolution. We decide to wait until we have an explanation for why things happen as they do. Until then, we use justification to rationalize how we behave around food.

Frustration and self-pity become energy, yielding to justifications. In relationships we often experience the behavior triangle, sometimes called the behavior triad. The three players in the relationship triad are the victim, the persecutor, and the rescuer. At any time the behavior can shift and the rescuer can become the victim, the victim can become the persecutor, and the persecutor can become the rescuer. All triangular behavior is about not being self-responsible. It is about the triangle.

After all these years working with people who are attached to food addictions, I have concluded that they play the triangle game within their own minds. Perhaps a painful life circumstance or some type of physical disability will lead them into the victim role. The internal rescuer will make allowances for them with food as reward. Soon the persecutor will get active and almost sound like the voice of an abuser. This all takes place in the mind. It is a mind triangle. It adds weight/wait.

So whenever you hear yourself saying things like "Oh, you can have just one. You deserve it." That is your rescuer playing to your victim. The victim sometimes says, "I just hurt so bad. I will just have what I want right now." The old persecutor will chastise you and get you to swear never to do it again, next week. Just wait.

## Why You Can't Have Your Cake & Eat It, Too

Expectations become justifications, which grow resentments. Resentments energize our victim, rescuer, and our persecutor. So we wait until we have the evidence our persecutor needs. We might wait until we have an understanding as to why things happen as they do. Our victim gains weight while he waits. It is an energetic logjam, bridge-out, or computer virus. These events are external, but they reflect the inner struggle. Soon we become the logjam. Try to remember the struggle is to let go of the blame game. The purpose of the blame game is to avoid personal responsibility for the choices we have made or the choices we need to make.

In an attempt to look at the ways you use expectations, resentments, and justifications, let's do an assessment. Get some quiet time and begin to journal on the following:

- What kind of situations do I find my self in repeatedly?

- What kind of people do I surround myself with constantly?

- How do I relate to myself? As victim, rescuer, or persecutor?

- How does that relationship change with different circumstances?

- What expectations do I have about money, jobs, relationships, love, and leisure time?

- What do I resent the most?

- What do I resent the least?

# Why You Can't Have Your Cake & Eat It, Too

After you get all of this down in black and white, read it out loud to yourself.  Listen.  Then when you feel ready to let all of these behaviors go, take your journal to the barbeque or fireplace.  By symbolically burning this old way of being, you are making your commitment to change.

## A Few Words About Ketosis

Those who attain ketosis often feel they have created a state of diet nirvana.   The truth is, ketosis is fat metabolism.  When fat is being oxidized, ketosis is taking place.  This is what we want to happen and is exactly the way the human body was engineered to work.  The human body is very adept at utilizing its fat.  Fat is the fuel the body wants to "burn".   It is stored in large deposits, and has a high energetic value.

Sugar prevents fat from being used as energy fuel because of its insulin requirement.   Remember, insulin is like the field commander on the battlefield.   Insulin takes first place in the hierarchy of usage.   It is like the boom box turned up to full volume.  It must be respected and listened to.  The processes of the body are tuned in to the signal of insulin.  Remember, it must be respected as the only hormone that responds to all sugar/carbohydrates in the diet.

The "ash" of fat oxidation is a ketone.  It is excreted through the skin and breath as a gas.  90% of ketones are released in the breath, and 10% in the stools and urine.  Give away those dip sticks!  You will know if you are in ketosis by the taste in your mouth and the fruity breath you will exude.

Most people in ketosis notice they are no longer hungry.  Amazingly, the swings of energy are no longer present.  There is a constant steady release of energy from your stored body fat.   Without the swings of energy that lead to fatigue, the stimulus for eating something to keep going is gone.   Your muscles do not go into fatigue or pain while you are burning fat. They are getting constant valuable fuel.

With the interference of carbohydrates, you become tired and hungry frequently.  Even with a good night's sleep, you might yawn, and then go to get some crackers or candy keep going. Ketosis is safe.   It is a part of the physiology created to use stored energy from fat reserves.   High carbohydrate eating disrupts this amazing process.

## A Few More Words

All of the information described in this plan is the result of my personal research and experience.  Each of you will find your own way to manage your food intake according to your lifestyle and the limits of your particular health needs.   Be gentle yet persistent with yourself as you begin to assemble all of the elements described.   Get started as soon as you can. The days of procrastination are ending.   Procrastination is weight and wait.

Protein-rich diets are often thought to be boring and not satisfying.  Many times I have seen longings for that certain something turned into a great new recipe.   I have seen patients make scrambled eggs taste like French toast. Lasagna and spaghetti have also been made using vegetables like zucchini as pasta. Ice cream has been made from Mori Nu Tofu and sugar free Jell-O.  Some of those recipes are included in this book.

# Why You Can't Have Your Cake & Eat It, Too

The items suggested here may not taste good to you, so in the beginning buy just the smallest amount to try. Willingness to keep trying new things will be a challenge that will yield great rewards. Adaptations can be made to create the taste and texture in foods to make them more desirable. Desserts can be found and made using high protein foods. This is a plan intended to last throughout life. Life is intended to last throughout the plan.

It has been calculated by researchers who have studied human metabolism that once the protein-to-carbohydrate-to-fat intake ratios are working properly, fat oxidation will proceed. Dr Flatt observed that if carbohydrate intake is restricted to less than 50 grams per day and protein consumption is at minimal levels (90 grams) then fat oxidation will proceed. He says it is possible to oxidize from 1/3 to 1/2 pound of fat per day. This represents 250 to 500 grams of body fat reserves used consistently. This is an average estimate.

Once the majority of the fluid retention is released, the typical fat loss will represent 2 to 3 pounds per week. George Blackburn, M.D. noted the progression of fluid loss in early fat reduction eating. Most of the fluids retained by the effects of hyperglycemia and hyper-insulinemia will be released during the first 3 weeks of low carbohydrate consumption. Many people who experience this loss at this time expect to lose this much weight every month. This initial fluid loss does not represent much fat loss. Body composition studies demonstrate this fact. This initiation loss is the water loss that precedes the use of fat.

# Why You Can't Have Your Cake & Eat It, Too

Consistent fat oxidation begins in the third week of low-carbohydrate-high-protein-moderate-fat diets.  It takes two to three weeks of corrective eating plans to dissipate the toxicity of hyperglycemia and hyper-insulinemia.  Individual variants will then come into play with fat loss results.  Some of these variables are seen in individual weight loss patterns.  While some people will lose the same amount week after week, others will lose in dribs and drabs for three weeks.  In the fourth week of the month, they will lose big.  It is like the big inning in a baseball game.  You wait and weight for the big inning, and suddenly there is the home run with the bases loaded.

Monthly hormonal patterns will create some fluid retention in some women.  By comparison, these fluid gains are nowhere near the fluid retention experienced in the high-carbohydrate days.  The intense cravings have also been diminished.  It is important to keep to the strategic eating plan during this time.  After the hormones have stabilized, the weight/wait loss rewards are great.  Hang in there.  It can and does happen.

Should the carbohydrate tolerances exceed the maximum levels, fat loss is much slower, if at all.  If carbohydrates are consumed late in the evening, overnight high blood sugar may stall out fat oxidation during the night.  Nighttime is fat-burning time.  Individuals will have sensitivity to carbohydrates based on genetics and physical symptoms that are inherent to them.  The 2 to 1 relationship of protein to carbohydrates typically will sustain fat oxidation levels because stored body fat is the fuel the body is burning.  This means the protein intake is at 100 grams per day and the carbohydrate intake is no more than 50 grams per day, for example.

## Why You Can't Have Your Cake & Eat It, Too

There are those who cannot tolerate 50 grams of carbohydrates a day due to physical disease and the length of time they have been above ideal body weight. They will need to have an eating strategy that will look like a 3 to 1 ratio of protein to carbohydrate. This represents 100 grams of protein to 35 grams of carbohydrate each day. Should the protein-to-carbohydrate intake ratio go to a 1 to 1 ratio (100 grams of protein and 100 grams of carbohydrate), weight loss will be much slower. Usually a carbohydrate increase of any amount will be detrimental to weight management and fat oxidation efforts.

Even if portions are cut below minimal levels, weight loss through fat oxidation will stall. This is that old portion control mentality rearing its ugly head one more time. Limiting all food, or fasting, or whatever one wants to call it, will not correct glucose toxicity or get fat loss going again. What is portion control? What would it look like? What foods would be limited and by how much? How much is too much? How much is too little. These are some of the important issues we need to understand. Portion control by way of restriction of protein, carbohydrates, and fat will stagnate fat loss. The danger in portion control and fasting is the body sacrificing its lean body mass for energy. These techniques will not work on weigh-in days at the clinic, either. I can tell if someone is fasting when they come in for a weigh-in appointment. It is part intuition and the other part blood pressure. Blood pressures are typically very low in fasting individuals. Fasting is a way of avoiding your results. It is a form of weight and wait, is it not?

Experience has been a good teacher, and it is important to apply the lesson to weight/wait management techniques.

# Why You Can't Have Your Cake & Eat It, Too

Wait is time.  Weight is gravity.  It has a way of growing.  It has a "weigh" of showing.

Drink your water.  Water intake is so important, and must be continued at all times.

## The Anatomy of Craving

Hungry, Angry, Lonely, Tired, and Scared= HALTS

These are some important directional signals capable of changing your relationship to food.  The words above describe some very significant states of feeling. Unscrambling your reactivity and resistance responses to these feelings will help you to strengthen your intuition. Personal insight is helpful in understanding your "need to feed".  It is said that we fight, flee, feed, or freeze when confronting something new or scary.  These words describe feeling/doing states that reflect themselves in resistance, reactance, and avoidance behaviors.  Improving your nutritional performance when exposed to these emotional signals is important.  I call it "weight/wait lifting".

Part of the improvement will be in the perceptions one has when in a difficult circumstance.  Someone has said that perception is everything - there is no reality.  Changing the way we look at a situation can be the impetus for changing the way we react, respond, or avoid it.  Truly the muscle needed to move us through life circumstances is the one of perceptions.  We tend to believe what we perceive.  It is possible then to change what one believes simply by changing what one perceives.  Some of us may call it turning a negative into a positive.  I call it research and development.

124

# Why You Can't Have Your Cake & Eat It, Too

It is lessons in learning. Being willing to look at the circumstances of life in a different way is often enough to change the energy of the reality.

The acronym "HALT" is well known as a "stop". (I added the "s" to add the emotion scared.) To my way of thinking the "halt" is a moment of willingness that one creates in order to re-perceive the circumstance. This is a moment of grace before intention is put into action. It is a gap in the timing mechanism of life. It allows one to see again. Look at it one more time and see if you see it the same way. When we are looking in a drawer full of objects for a special screwdriver, how often do we slam it shut, thinking someone has borrowed it and not returned it? We start imagining all kinds of ways to get even for this infraction. We may even begin to prepare a speech to deliver to the "thief." Then from some little quiet voice we hear, "Why don't you look in that drawer again?" And so we do. There it is, the screwdriver, exactly where it belonged.

Thankfully this moment of willingness gave you the ladder to get off of your high horse. Halt is meant to stop. It just happens that the letters that form the word are the first letters of feeling words. Seeing the situation in a different way is to develop one's awareness in the possibility of choice.

It is one thing to smell the rose. It is quite another thing to see it. Let's go through some of these important feeling words. Let us look at them again with fresh eyes.

# Why You Can't Have Your Cake & Eat It, Too

## Hunger

Hunger is a part of the stomach, blood sugar, and brain loop. As the nutrients in the blood supply begin to decrease, the brain begins its signaling to the stomach. The stomach begins to feel empty. and may even growl. We then look for something to eat. If we are angry, we feed it. If we are scared we freeze it, usually with ice cream. If we are scared, we flee it, usually with chocolate. If we are lonely, we fight it with popcorn. These feeling states put us close to feeding states.

A part of our cultural rules dictates when we are supposed to eat. The collective mind will also tell us the foods we are to consume at a particular mealtime. Eggs and cereal are to be eaten at breakfast. If someone suggests a breakfast of tuna salad and cottage cheese, then such words as "outrageous" come to mind. Often we are told to eat when we are hungry. This may mean we will need to eat something every 2 to 3 hours. Again and again the judgment police will tell you, "You can't eat that way!" In an effort to gain approval, we may postpone eating something until it is that "time". We may put our needs down, to please someone else. It never works. When the time does come to nourish ourselves, we often over consume many foods.

## Nurturance and nourishment represent ways to refuel our lives.

Each of us has a unique hunger personality, so it makes sense that each of us gets hungry at different times. Your personal hunger message needs to be acknowledged as soon as possible. We can predict the times of day we will need to eat if we are paying attention to our feeling states. The spiritual masters teach, "Eat when hungry, and sleep when tired." Often while we are "waiting" to eat, we get overly hungry. This type of hunger is very hard to withstand.

Having a "911" kit of back-up protein-rich foods will be helpful at times like these. This would mean that you keep on hand high-protein snacks or drinks that can be eaten quickly. Is a nearby restaurant available capable of preparing a protein meal for you? These snacks could also be consumed as prevention before we are overwhelmed with hunger.

Then there are the times when we completely go off our plan. Perhaps there is more alcohol intake. Surely the carbohydrate intake goes off the charts. This will cause extreme cravings as you attempt to regain your sense of direction. During this phase, go to a complete protein diet --- an entire day of protein. Consuming 2 or 3 ounces of protein every 2 to 3 hours will give you the power to handle the surges of hunger. Be sure to include enough protein to reach your daily intake goal. This technique can be helpful to jump-start the diet after a trip, or after a binge. Remember, you can't control the setback, but you can control yourself.

Time has a way of getting a way from us, or so we say. Preparation is an important measure of the time you have. The time you have is important to measure.

## Anger

This is a very high voltage feeling. It has its roots in fear and control. For our purposes, it is important to acknowledge anger's role in the development of the need to consume a substance. Sometimes we feel the need to get even, extract revenge, teach someone a lesson, portray the martyr, or even the score.   Where the break occurs is when we believe we are powerless to be heard.  Some of us implode. Some of us explode.   It is important to accept how ineffective these strategies are in managing anger.   Eating over it, chewing someone out, having someone for lunch, and stuffing it are some interesting terms we use to describe some actions taken around anger.

What to do?  Acknowledge your anger.  Then trace it back to its root emotion, fear.   I define fear, as "False evidence appears real."   Look again at the object of your frustration. Ask yourself, "Does this action nourish my soul, or does it serve my need to be right?"   Feeding your anger is like "Taking poison and hoping someone else dies."

Often anger comes from a perceived lack of control over a person, place or a situation.  Should the delicate balance of power one is trying to impose become unbalanced, the controlling person gets out of control.   Anger is a state of being that is often exhibited in proportion to the perception of a lack of control.  Controlling people are the most scared.  It does not appear that way, because angry people do not create sympathy for themselves.   Most angry people find themselves being avoided, when they really crave friendship.

Angry, controlling people are the most scared.  Fear, anger, and control are part of a negative attractor pattern.  These states of being do not support life or wellness.  In support of life and the mission to recover wellness, choice is going to be a crucial factor for you.   Choosing indulgence or choosing intelligence is up to you.   In making a decision the most important factor is intention, which incorporates a state of

128

being in contemplation of taking action.  Consider an intention like acceptance or willingness.  Opposite this type of positive intention is revenge or depression.  Intention is important.  It is behind the choices we make.

While it might appear as though they eat their young, an angry person is really trying to keep people from abandoning them.  It is said that we attract what we fear, and then it is possible to push people away by controlling behaviors.

To be on the receiving end of an angry, controlling person is a very unsettling experience.  Angry outbursts are meant to take away your power.  It follows, then, to see victims of anger or abuse feed themselves with comfort foods in an effort to restore the power they gave up to their abuser.  In fact, many times the victim has retreated from the angry person, but he takes on further abuse with life-desecrating behaviors.  In many cases he will pick on himself just as his abuser did.

In working groups or in the workplace, we are seeing and experiencing unprecedented hostility.  A pecking order develops around the perception of oppression, whether real or imagined.  Sometimes working groups feel oppressed by the institution or by the hand life has dealt them.  This oppression shows itself in the workplace as co-workers become intolerant and even abusive to one another.  Similar behaviors have been noted in gangs, prison populations, and slaves.  A power hierarchy is developed, and those in the working environment know who to side with or who to isolate.  The women's movement has often decried the glass ceiling as an imposed boundary established by the male business mentality.  This excuse is just a distraction from the real infighting that goes on between women in the workplace.

# Why You Can't Have Your Cake & Eat It, Too

As hard as it is, it is vital to look at anger as fear.  It takes just a moment of willingness to shift the hold anger has on our behavior.  Even to address the anger as a friend calling us to examine the thing we fear the most is a change in perception.  You may not get to the bottom line of your fear, but you did change the way you related to it.  This is a good beginning.  Try to remember that you always have a choice and that you matter.

## Loneliness

Companionship is particularly important in our human development.  There are countless studies demonstrating the importance of human connectedness.  Isolation or feeling unwanted are infectious organisms in the perception we call loneliness.  Celebrations call for family and friends to gather around the table.  Sharing common stories feeds the soul, and sharing common foods feed the body.  When we are alone there is no one to share our food or our experience.  Eating, feeding, and over-consuming is common when we feel we are not appreciated.  The need to fill up the empty space is often the impetus for the urge to splurge.  Missing out on some experience, feeling left out or abandoned, we may try to sweeten our sour mood with food.  We may even believe no one will care if we gain a few more pounds.  After all is said and done, no one cares.

Combating loneliness is a proactive effort.  It requires a deep commitment to be what you want to attract.  It is an inside job.  Learning ways to calm yourself without a substance or addictive habit will pay huge dividends.  Journaling, meditation, volunteering, and calling a friend are ways to address one's loneliness. Learning to be a friend to yourself is the difficult task, is it not? Craving companionship is a human need. We are not meant to be alone. Yet we stuff the need for meaningful human connections, displacing our loneliness with foods. Calming oneself can be done without an attachment to a substance. It requires training just like any skill we want to develop.

Growing through our experiences is a part of the process that makes us available to be a friend to others. Mother Teresa said that the greatest pain in the world was caused by the inability to sit and be silent. Time alone can be a gift. Privacy is an important boundary, and all of us need it in small amounts. Yet we find ourselves longing for companionship, even romance. Some of us know our restaurant servers better than we know our neighbors. We need to address our own personal behaviors when we are trying to figure out why we don't have friends or love in our life.

Not too many years ago, one of my clients was bemoaning the fact that she had been single for twenty years. What really irked her was that she had lost over 100 pounds and still could not attract a partner. Before I gave her my impression, I couched my remarks by reminding her how much I loved her. I then reminded her that the reason she had not found love in her life was that she simply was not ready for it yet. The Universe had a bigger plan for her. I also reminded her about the principle of attraction. This meant her negativity was a repellant. Many times we are alone because we need to work on our negative mental attitudes and the sense of entitlement they generate. Happily, she worked on her belief systems. She found that smiling was an exercise that generated a strong magnetic attraction. Getting out of her own drama, she began to allow herself to be available to make conversation with others that wasn't about her. She started shopping for new clothes, and changed her makeup. Suddenly she noticed she felt attracted to a man and he seemed especially interested in her. This relationship grew into love. It took time. It was worth the wait.

When fat is used as a protector, it can be scary to lose the sense of false security it symbolizes. This protection can act as an insulator or a barrier. As different levels of weight are lost from the body, there can be flashbacks to times when one was at that weight in another experience. This may generate the need to isolate once more by applying the brakes to the weight loss. This braking symbolizes wait, weight. It is a stop. These are moments when we may sabotage ourselves with negative repeating behaviors. Negative repeating behaviors are simply research and development. These times present themselves so we can learn to recognize the elements that create self-sabotage.

Self-sabotage is always about fear. When the human body is approaching an ideal size, then one may lose the sense of protection that fat symbolized. While the sense of protection existed, it was also as an illusion. The painful experience that created this need to be protected and to be isolated is no longer present. Yet the body retains this experience in its cellular memory. As this moment comes into your awareness, just the thought of being available to the possibility of this kind of painful experience causes you to go into the illusion of protection and control.

The physical barriers seem to be the easiest to remove. The mental and soul barriers challenge us the most. Removing our barriers to becoming a full-fledged member of the human race means letting go of the resistance we have to go with the flow. Yes, here is resistance once more. Our physical resistance is often a mirror of our intellectual and spiritual resistance. The inside shows up on the outside. It has wait and weight.

Here is a prayer for healing loneliness:

"Life is so generous a giver, but we, judging its gifts by their covering, cast them away as ugly or heavy, or hard. Remove the covering, and you will find beneath it a living splendor, woven of love, by wisdom, with power.

"Welcome it, grasp it, and you will touch the angel's hand that brings it to you. Everything we call a trial, a sorrow or a duty, believe me, that angel's hand is there; the gift is there, and the wonder of an overshadowing presence. Our joys, too: be not content with them as joys. They too conceal diviner gifts.

"And so, at this time I greet you. Not quite as the world sends greetings, but with profound esteem, and with the prayer that for you now and forever, the day breaks, and the shadows flee".

Fra Giovanni

## Tiredness

When do you get tired? Where does your fatigue appear in your body? Do you postpone getting the needed rest? Do you see yourself feeding your fatigue with constant snacking? Honestly answering those questions will give you cues demonstrating where and how you manage your physical energy.

Sometimes our eyes get tired. Others complain of muscle aches. These are subtle energy clues reminding us to take time to rest. Eating through fatigue is a losing proposition. Usually high carbohydrate foods are selected and used in large quantities. It doesn't take too long to feel the effects of lots of sugar. The resulting overload yields the toxic reaction you know so well. The swings of energy, up and down, are exhausting. This compounds the existing fatigue.

It takes discipline to commit to getting adequate rest and relaxation. Sleep is a fat-burning activity. It is during the hours of sleep that the body goes to its fat reserves for energy. The benefits of getting a good night's rest are better than any pill or substance. Become familiar with your limits. The healthy glow following a good night is an obvious sign of good health. What are you weighting/waiting for?

There is an epidemic of fatigue growing in our collective bodies today. There is also an epidemic of muscle fatigue in proportion to the energetic fatigue in this disease relationship. The diagnostic term used to describe this phenomenon is Chronic Fatigue Syndrome and Fibromyalgia. These terms denote profound states of fatigue and muscle inertia. It is a startling coincidence that the majority of those so diagnosed are many pounds over their ideal body size, and present with many of the symptoms of insulin resistance.

I saw a patient who was 120 pounds over her ideal body weight. It was an extreme effort for her to move from the car into any location for any purpose. It took much energy for her to work or to care for herself.  She also had sleep apnea, so it was impossible for her to sleep the whole night through.  The exhaustion came first, and then the muscles gave in as well. Bearing so much extra weight is a serious strain on the muscle groups.  Combined with the insulin resistance, the muscle fibers were unable to get vital nutrients from the process of nutrition.

Here is the formula for the cycle of fatigue:

Sleep Apnea
Plus
Insulin Resistance
Plus
Large Fat Reserves
Yields
Chronic Fatigue and Fibromyalgia

Supplying a corrective nutritional strategy to relieve insulin resistance will at once improve Fibromyalgia. Lots of protein and lots of water are needed to feed those hungry hurting muscles.  Starving muscles will find nutrients from the ample fatty acids.   As fat reserves are utilized for energy, the energetic highs and lows level out, for it is no longer necessary to get energy from dietary sugar.  As the weight of fat is relinquished from the muscles, pain is lessened.  Then as the large visceral fat mass that impinges on the diaphragm is relinquished, the sleep apnea is relieved and the natural sleep cycle is restored.   The fat pad in the back of the throat that used to contribute to the sleep apnea is also removed by fat oxidation.

# Why You Can't Have Your Cake & Eat It, Too

The following are some very wise words discussing how simple the solutions can be to our seemingly complex problems. We have over-analyzed and pathologized the need to get a good night's sleep and lose weight.

"Our true home is in the present moment. To live in the present moment is a miracle. The miracle is not to walk on water. The miracle is to walk on the green Earth in the present moment, to appreciate the peace and beauty that are available now. Peace is all around us, in the world and in nature, within us, in our bodies and our spirits. Once we learn to touch this peace, we will be healed and transformed. It is not a matter of faith; it is a matter of practice".

Thich Nhat Hanh

## Fear

Fear is the thief that keeps on stealing. It steals our confidence and seals our fate. Each one of us has a fear that pushes all the wrong buttons, yet we invite it in every chance. Fear of the unknown, public speaking, getting sick, getting healthy, and on and on the list goes. If this is your issue, there is a super book by Robert Gerzon called, <u>Finding Serenity in the Age of Anxiety.</u> Read it.

For our understanding, it is important to note how strongly fear commands our life. This is especially true when we are anxious. While it would be great if we could all feel safe, it is not the case. Sometimes eating over fear is one of the most out of control experiences we face.

## Why You Can't Have Your Cake & Eat It, Too

Try to step out of the situation and look at yourself while you are engaging in your habit.   This is a time when you should see yourself with compassion.   Developing compassion for your suffering through fear, you might also become aware of the attachment placed on food when one is in the experience of fear.   You may not be anywhere near the person, place or thing that scares you.   You may only have a memory or a flashback to a trauma.   Yet, you and I are so willing to pick up the lash where our abusers left it last.   We give ourselves a whipping when no one is around when we engage in negative self-harming behaviors.   These may be bulimia, cutting, or stuffing.   These experiences give us an illusion of control.

The person who is the most frightened is usually the most controlling. This is one of the rules of the universe.   As you experience fear and the controlling behaviors can you see yourself with compassion?

It is a paradox that we fear getting healthy and taking the steps to succeed.   How can we fear such a positive outcome?   It is because we know we can succeed, and this terrifies us.   Think how often we see self-sabotage.   Our succeeding may mean accepting our changing physiologic picture.   It may mean we go it alone.   While this fear rarely materializes, we may fantasize all kinds of scenarios. Holidays, celebrations, and vacations involve food.   What will happen?

Here is an action list:

Choosing not to choose is a choice.

Create your life with abundant choices.

# Why You Can't Have Your Cake & Eat It, Too

Never underestimate how strong, flexible, and creative you are.

Try to keep a stash of safe high protein foods that can be used when you become fearful or out of control.

Call someone.  Let them know that you need their help. Call me.

Ask yourself where it is in your body you feel the fear. This subtle signal will redirect you.

Today you have a life full of choices.  The most frightening thing is to lose the ability to choose.  When you are overweight, with many of the illnesses that are associated with insulin resistance, your choices are very limited and the choices you have are not the ones you want.  The identity you are creating is created out of the choices you make.  They show.  What you do in private shows up in public.  Fear is not the private experience we would like it to be.  The mysteries of life can be a challenge.   The next two writings are words of comfort.   They have comforted me, and I hope they will comfort you.

From A Course In Miracles (Text, page 188)

"What is healing but the removal
Of all that stands in the way of knowledge?
And how else can one dispel illusions
Except by looking at them directly,
Without protecting them?
Be not afraid, therefore,
For what you will be looking at

# Why You Can't Have Your Cake & Eat It, Too

Is the source of fear
And you are beginning to learn
That fear is not real".

And…..

"You are so young, so before all beginning, and I want to beg you, as much as I can, to be patient toward all that is unsolved in your heart and to try to love the questions themselves like the locked rooms and like books that are written in a very foreign tongue.

"Do not now seek the answers, which cannot be given you because you would not be able to live them.  And the point is, to love everything.  Live the questions now.  Perhaps you will then gradually, without noticing it, live along some distant day into the answer".

Rainer Maria Rilke

## Boredom

Believe it or not, boredom is about perfection and inertia working together.  When we are bored, we usually sigh meaninglessly and do absolutely nothing.  Boredom is the result of the need to maintain a level of perfection.  Since the perfection is illusive, the imaginary sense of control is never achieved.  Then inertia sets in, going nowhere very slowly.  Bored people are demanding and temperamental.  This is an example of the rocket on the launch pad running a full load of fuel, with no intention of lifting off.  They wait.  We weight.

# Why You Can't Have Your Cake & Eat It, Too

As problematic as perfectionism can be, so is the inertia. There seems to be a problem with making commitments of any kind. It is waiting. The distant day never comes when you are living in the future. It is hard to get around a perfectionist.

Another look at the perfectionist reveals someone who is afraid to fail - whatever that means. So they don't even try. It then becomes a cycle of not participating in life, lack of commitment, and waiting. Yes, boredom is about fear. Let us look at the accumulators. These are people that are unable to get rid of their old stuff. The fears that drive hoarding are many. They can be about the fear of scarcity, approval fears, or the fear losing something important. The clutter of accumulation may be so great, the chaos so powerful; our accumulator is ground into total inertia.

This is true of the issue with morbid obesity. Here the accumulation is so great, that our accumulator is hopelessly mired. The chaotic health drama may be unfolding like Mr. Toad's wild ride. The issues of daily living are in a perpetual state of meltdown. Going nowhere, gaining weight, and feeling sick.

Boredom can trigger cravings and hunger. It is very insidious due to its subtle, albeit sneaky, appearance. Things may be going along very well. The pink cloud phase of your diet may be waning. You are eating the same food plan repeatedly. It gets boring. Change is good, provided it is good change. But before that change happens, the craving cycle gets activated. Check yourself out for food boredom. You may say, "I must be doing something wrong." The most likely scenario is you are eating the same thing, fixed the same way each and every day.  Keeping the diet fresh and new is very important.  The human palate likes change.  In fact, the word palate (palette) is used to describe a surface on which one applies color to create a painting.  The human palate is a surface on which to create changes.  Changing the tea bags for your ice tea, using different vegetables, and varying protein types will give you the sense of relief you are looking for from this type of hunger.  The rule of paradox is a part of the boredom and perfection behavior.  Again, we attract what we fear.  Fears of scarcity, approval, and of giving away something important function here.  Health becomes scarce.  Disapproval is rampant for those who are morbidly obese.  And yes, something important is given away- self worth.

"Nightmares are not real. "
Mister Rogers

## Chapter Four:
## The Cultural Mind

### A little bit of history

A long time ago,  early humans used their stores of body fat to survive.    This survival fat was stored body fat they accumulated  from fat sources in their diet.  There is no doubt early man had encountered many difficult experiences. Not only did he have to outrun ferocious beasts and other enemies, but  he also had to carry water, hunt for food, make shelters, provide clothing, and travel vast distances in search of suitable climates.  It is estimated that early man and woman used 15,000 calories a day. Today, by contrast, the Recommended Daily Allowance(RDA) in calories, as calculated on the food pyramid, is 2,400-3000 calories per day.

While none of us normal civilians can imagine working that hard, it is important to visualize what kind of workload our early native people endured.   A professional football player will expend 5,000 calories per hour of continuous play.  A professional basketball player will most likely expend approximately the same amount of calories per hour.   The quantity of water needed to support that kind of activity is also a very important source of energy.

Another factor in our survival is our ability to reproduce.  We see in our starving populations today high rates of infant mortality and infertility.  In our anorexic humans, we see the same kind of statistics.   But there are more surprises in our obese and insulin-resistant humans; they too struggle with infertility and infant mortality.    Human fat stores create estrogen.   This constant insulin suppresses the hormones necessary for fertility in both men and women.  This is seen in the feminizing effect obesity has on men.

This factor is distressing, but in women there is another interesting development.  It is known that insulin stimulates the ovaries.   An over-secretion of insulin, however, will suppress the ovaries, leading to the problem of polycystic ovarian syndrome.    The insulin suppression of the ovary leads to the overproduction of testosterone.  The testosterone has a negative impact on the ovary, leading to cyst formation, infertility, and suppression of menses.

As difficult as the concept may be for you to grasp,, try to accept the idea that having fat stores is a good thing. Remember, stored fat represents usable high energy.  Stored fat is the body's preferred energy source.  Getting fat into energy mode is how we are wired.  With the eating strategy suggested here, you will slowly move significant amounts of fat into energetic production.  This will put you into a ketone-burning state.  Because you are keeping your blood sugar low, you will not be creating a harmful back-up of blood gases. That condition, which we see in out-of-control high blood sugar, is called keto-acidosis, and it involves rapid destruction of living tissues, requiring swift intervention.

## Feast and Famine

The feast-and-famine theory of fat regulation worked for our ancestors.  In the evolution of humanity, it appears that our ability to store fat continues to this day.  Our one big problem is the inability to mobilize our fat stores for use on a daily basis. A pound of body fat contains 3,500 calories. This represents energy -- fuel for the activities of daily living. Imagine our fat reserves as an energetic fuel tank. Unfortunately, for many this fuel tank is inaccessible. Access to it is blocked, in part due to genetic factors and in part due to the high-carbohydrate low-fat manner by which we feed ourselves today.

Unrestricted access to carbohydrate-rich nutrients inhibits fat oxidation. Carbohydrates must be used first, due to the high-priority pancreatic insulin response. The insulin response in combination with the carbohydrate-rich diet we now consume makes consistent fat oxidation impossible. Insulin tells your body that food is plentiful; therefore it is not necessary to oxidize the stored fat. When insulin is in charge, so to speak, it uses a boom-box turned to high volume to convey its message, to insure that it will not be ignored.

Metabolically speaking, we are constructed to burn or oxidize our stores of fat on a consistent basis. Fat is a preferred fuel type with the highest possible fuel rating, and it accumulates in astonishing progression. This is apparent in the American eating culture. The low-fat eating we have been doing for the past thirty years has created obesity in sad and staggering statistics. This public health crisis will not go away with portion control, exercise, and will power. We must reduce the insulin response and the only way to do that is to reduce the intake of carbohydrates.

We are like rockets on launch pads, revving our engines, but not burning the highest-octane fuel. It is this constant revving that wears down the immune system, pancreas, kidneys, gastrointestinal function, and cardiovascular systems.

# Why You Can't Have Your Cake & Eat It, Too

Cardiovascular irritation, slowed gastric emptying, chronic fatigue, adult-onset diabetes, peripheral vascular meltdown, kidney impairment --- is there need for any more evidence? These are the results of prolonged high blood sugar and high blood insulin.

Metaphorically speaking, as a culture we are in the famine cycle. Our unique prosperity has created a type of malnutrition. In the this current form of starvation, our bodies are being destroyed, bit by bit, as we try to outlast prolonged high blood sugar and prolonged high blood insulin. Our body is also chronically dehydrated and protein-deprived. This age of malnutrition is the result of the culture of endless consumerism, without one thought given as how to pay for the things we consume. The "Have now, pay later" culture causes debt in both realms, metaphysical and physical.

Storing fat is a normal function. It insured that our early humans could survive long periods of deprivation. Using stored fat is a normal function, but to use stored fat certain conditions must be present. The foremost condition is to reduce the need for pancreatic insulin. This will enable the body to move fat from the storage compartment into the metabolic nuclear reactor.

## Low Fat Ground Zero

About sixty years ago the Second World War ended and the Armed Forces came home to unprecedented prosperity. Television was now available in the home. The automobile became the transportation of choice. The fast food industry was just getting under way. Many labor-saving inventions were available for use in many ways. Travel, leisure time, and convenience were expected.  The culture of the time placed value on hard work and ingenuity.  What would the price of these new opportunities be in terms of physical health and well being?

Somewhere in the collective mind there existed a belief system. Work and inventiveness were associated with being healthy.  Prosperity and lack of activity were seen associated with royalty. With unrestricted access to plentiful food and less activity associated with the automobile, wouldn't we get fat? Didn't the wealthy become inactive and therefore practice gluttony?  Was it possible that on a smaller scale each family could become its own form of royalty with this new culture of prosperity?  Those minds concerned with public health began to manipulate the health future of America.  Could this great land become a wasteland of hopelessly obese couch potatoes?  There was so much concern about possible mass obesity that a study was begun under the direction of Alan Stunkard, M.D. a Pennsylvania psychiatrist.

The determinations made by Stunkard and his team insured that we would all turn out just as we feared -- obese couch potatoes.  A one-generational rat study was put in place. Yes, rats.  We know much more about animals today than we know about humans.  These little creatures were put in cages (of course), fed lots of food, and given no exercise. Someone may have exposed them to television.  It didn't take too long for the results to come in.  The rats got fat!

The conclusion reached by the Stunkard study was: if you eat too much of everything and don't exercise you will get fat. This created the belief system or belief program, which drives the weight loss industry, the exercise industry, the food manufacturers, the federal government, and professional nutritional education systems. Coincidental to this conclusion was the existent cultural belief system: prosperity creates a fat leisure class. As the results were made known there was a collective sigh of relief from the food manufacturers. No one was singled out for wrongdoing. They were all wrong, if you will. So if you are all wrong then you are all included in the solution.

The next question was, "Well, what do we do about it?" Since no one was going to be excluded, everything would be included. The concepts of smaller portions of everything, lots of exercise, and the old "Calories-in must equal calories-out" theory of weight management was the conclusion of the nutritional studies done on the rats. These were experimental conclusions, with liberal preferences given to the important food industry. Most importantly, it supported the old belief system of wealth breeding a fat leisure class. If these theories would be put into practice, we could be saving humanity from becoming overfat. We were told we could have what we wanted as long as we controlled our portions and exercised. There would be no restrictions put on any product.

Putting this theory into practice would require a little more will power than previously needed in all of World War II. The "greatest generation" was now being challenged by a mythical foe more terrible than war: an obese leisure class. Little was heard or known about insulin and its impact on physiological functioning. Today we have thin, hard-working people who have evolved into the diseases that used to afflict only the obese. Hard work, portion control, and now will power would have no power on insulin resistance.

# Why You Can't Have Your Cake & Eat It, Too

The food pyramid with its layers of commercial distraction was instituted. In fact, the food pyramid has become its own institution. It has become the touch point for food labeling, government-sponsored feeding programs, and the famous "recommended daily allotments" for food intake. It represents the high carbohydrate, low protein, low fat eating style that has driven us into the obesity we now have. But for exercise, the critics argue, we wouldn't get fat.

Weight loss gadgets made millionaires out of their inventors. Diet books with diet foods created millionaires, as did diet clubs and commercial diet plans. The exercise industry got going and created millions for their entrepreneurs. Unfortunately, obesity kept going. It seemed to be unstoppable. If all of these things worked, then how did the population continue to get fat? Thigh Master? Nordic Track? Could the problem be with food intake?

Many people argued about this question. In fact today, almost everybody has a closely-held belief system about the meaning of "diet". Ninety-nine per cent of the time, when the question is raised about losing weight, the sound level in the room will begin to elevate. Everyone has a theory and a belief system that drives it. Diets have become their own icons.

The designation of food groups was meant to distract us from the chemistry of food. Shifting nutritional labels further obscure our vision for food values. New food adjectives with a medicinal sound are difficult to understand or put into practical use. Nutria-cuticals anyone? These food categories and special designations have just one purpose -- to distract and deter any meaningful discussion specific to food and how the human body functions with this important fuel.

## Why You Can't Have Your Cake & Eat It, Too

Additionally, these labels and designations are used in the service of protection for the great yet fragile food industry.

The food pyramid was meant to set the standard for acceptable human nutrition.  The reality is, the food pyramid gave the food industry equal representation in the market place.   Recently we have seen such terms as the glycemic index, complex food, organic, natural, low carb, and healthy used to describe a food type.   The words good and bad cannot be used to describe food.  The protectionist food lobby has even instituted a law that makes it an offense to denigrate a food.   However, if you were fat, you were thought to be bad. If you were thin, then you were good.   There are no laws to regulate that.

The results of the rodent studies of the '50's are still being applied to the circumstances we find today in our society. Food protectionism is still in force.   Commercial weight loss plans, gym memberships, and health food trickery are adding more insult to the gathering disaster of overwhelming obesity and insulin resistance.   The key point is insulin resistance., which can occur in normal-weighted non-obese people, but It always occurs in obesity.

Here is a short list of the belief systems related to nutrition. Which of these or other belief systems have  you incorporated into your nutritional programming?   Remember, these ideas were experimental, with no input from human laboratory studies.  For the intention of observation only, think of these things as delusional!   They are examples of intellectual resistance.

# Why You Can't Have Your Cake & Eat It, Too

- Exercise gives weight loss

- Sugar causes weight gain

- Inactivity causes weight gain

- Unlimited access to food will cause obesity

- Will power is the key to weight management

- Eat the food pyramid & but control those portions

The food producers are subsidizing the American Heart Association and the American Diabetic Association. This fact has the appearance of selling out the best interest of the community for the bottom line in these industries. The food pyramid is based on recommendations from the USDA, who answers to the food lobby. The USDA recommends much less protein per kilogram of ideal body weight than is found in the scientific literature. There is a tremendous amount of wheeling and dealing taking place between the food industry and the not-for-profit health organizations. These deals provide for hefty payments to the ADA and the AHA for product endorsement.

You will have to be your own best bodyguard when it comes to marketing. The government will not protect us from unscrupulous claims from nutritional supplements, nor from advertising claims.

# Why You Can't Have Your Cake & Eat It, Too

## A new light

Approximately thirty years later, some new light was being reflected on the emerging obesity epidemic. A couple of medical doctors were looking at the increasing numbers of chronic diseases in their obese populations. They noted primarily that the obesity factor was always present with the conditions of high blood pressure, adult-onset diabetes, high cholesterol, and coronary artery disease. In other words, if someone was overweight, their chances of becoming chronically ill were great. There was a connection, but it was not fully understood. Gerald Reaven was one of the men who began to connect the metabolic dots. It was a slow process, but it was a beginning.

In the late 1970's Dr Reaven gave a famous lecture at Banting in which he noted these concurrent health conditions. He coined the term the "the deadly quartet" for them, since these conditions would lead to the demise of the patient. Later this became a syndrome with the ominous-sounding name: "Metabolic Syndrome X" or if you prefer, "Reaven's Syndrome". In later years he expanded this syndrome to include gout, family history of non-insulin-dependent diabetes mellitus, gastro-esophageal reflux, irritable bowel syndrome, and an abdominal circumference greater than 30 inches for a woman or 38 inches for a man. Remember, these conditions indicated that the individual would go on to develop "Reaven's Syndrome". Later he would inform us that the causative factor in this metabolic syndrome was insulin resistance. It was becoming apparent that it was the body's own defensive response to insulin that was driving the disorders of obesity.

# Why You Can't Have Your Cake & Eat It, Too

Many questions remained unanswered, but one thing remained constant. Obesity continued to grow. To be sure portion control, calorie counting and exercise were implemented in the suggested care of these patients. It rarely worked.

In the very late 1980s there was a very important double-blind study performed on human subjects. For the first time in recorded history humans were studied in relationship to nutrients in food. Dr.Flatt wrote and researched extensively on human use and storage of nutrients. He still conducts research today, and his writings are very illuminative, shedding new light on nutrient usage by humans. His papers conclude that the old belief systems represent a type of nutritional mythology and have no basis in real human physiologic functioning.

Here is a short list of some of his conclusions in human nutritional physiology:

- Carbohydrates must be used first

- Carbohydrates can be stored in limited amounts as glycogen and tryglycerides

- Carbohydrates will become a type of fat when the fat intake falls below 10 grams per day

- Carbohydrates require insulin

- Protein and fat do not require insulin

- Protein cannot be stored

# Why You Can't Have Your Cake & Eat It, Too

- Protein must be re-supplied each day

- Fat is preferred fuel

- Fat is always stored

As I read this important work, I began to see how selectively conditioned we have become as consumers. The illusions about food, exercise, and weight management techniques have created this epidemic of obesity. We will not be able to work our way out of it with portion control or exercise. We will have to scrutinize the types of food we now have in our diet. We did not come with a scanner implanted in the stomach. At some point we are going to have to come to terms with that approach when someone says a particular food is this or that.

We can see how persuasive the collective mind has been in dictating how we continue to behave around nutrients. Artificial sweeteners have been developed and put in food. This nourished the belief that you could have your cake and eat it, too. Today it looks as though that won't work, either. When the fat-blocking drug hit the street, there was a cadre of doctors pushing it at the behest of the drug companies. Didn't anyone notice that it was carbohydrates that the population is addicted to? No matter that the fat-blockers gave nasty unpleasant, unpredictable oily bowel movements. The FDA did ban the carbohydrate-blocking drugs, but the health food companies have created their own version of hope in a bottle and it doesn't work, either.

We will have to make a concession to the idea that the chemistry of nutrients and genetics dictates the human body's ability to utilize nutrients. We must abandon the portion-control- exercise mentality that has created this public health crisis we know as obesity.  We must abandon the fat-free eating programs that continue to drive this epidemic to its logical conclusion before it  cripples two-thirds or more of the adults in America.  We are all going to die, but will we become a nation of dead men and women walking?

 Will we continue to perform punishing exercise routines with the expectation we will get weight loss?  Often injuries occur and we give up.  When there is significant obesity it makes sense that the feet, legs, back, and hips will carry the stress of intense workouts. There will be pain, and then  gain, if we deny into oblivion that carbohydrates are both the cause and the cure for controlling insulin-resistance and any meaningful weight management.

Obesity and its cascading health problems are in epidemic proportions.  The effects of this epidemic are yet to be realized.  As the population ages, the health-related consequences will be felt in many agonizing ways.  These consequences have the potential to cripple families, the community, and the country financially.

In a way, obesity is a form of serious malnutrition, and  this malnutrition needs to be addressed by a paradigm shift in our collective nutritional  mind.  It is plain to see that the old paradigm is not working for us, for its results are all around us. The old paradigm hasn't worked and it won't work now because of the evolution of human beings.  We see in family histories that adult-onset diabetes is striking our youngsters. High cholesterol levels are now found in 20-year-olds.  Our human insulin resistance is increasing with exposure and time. We will constantly have to shift our carbohydrate intake to match our changing immunity to insulin.

Florence Nightingale was a keen observer of public health issues. When the clergy of her day endorsed prayer and church attendance as a way to combat the cholera epidemic affecting London at the time, Miss Nightingale was highly irritated. She dismissed this religious solution as nonsense. She is reported to have said that the swamps need to be drained and the gutters cleared in order for the community to be relieved of cholera.

Symbolically speaking, this is what we need to do. We need to address the issues that no longer work in controlling this health crisis. Then we need to replace them with sound nutritional principles coming out of the human studies on nutrition. There can be no sacred cows of old thinking or protective economic coddling. This crisis needs to be taken seriously, now.

Most of the storage of body fat in today's humans is located around the circumference of the belly button. This fat is also called visceral fat, because of its location in and around the internal organs. It is known that abundant body fat is stored in this location, and also that this fat is extremely insulin-resistant. This fat begins the auto-immune response to carbohydrates and insulin and sensitizes the body to become "allergic" to the effects of insulin.

This is a part of the "why'" we have become insulin-resistant. Remember, if you have a family history of coronary artery disease, gout, high blood pressure, adult onset diabetes, and high cholesterol you are at risk of becoming insulin-immune.

## Chapter Five
## The Elephant in the Treatment Room

## Symptom Based Treatment

From prehistoric man to today's man, there has been a wide swing in our evolutionary abilities. Gaining mastery over the environment, inventing many new technologies, and learning new methods has exposed the world we know to constant and unrelenting change. The ability to store fat has been the factor which helped insure the survival of our species. When all else failed, stored body fat helped humankind endure. Today our body fat has just the opposite effect. It has crippled us in the obvious ways of appearance and mobility. The destruction of health may not be as obvious, but surely obesity has exacted a terrific toll on this aspect of life. The economic impact of obesity is just now being evaluated. Days off work, prescription drugs, and health insurance premiums are some examples of the cost of this very personal problem.

Long ago I was a part of developing a care strategy for a patient, beginning with a round table discussion with all of the practitioners who might have some influence on the outcome of this individual. Data were presented relating to age, height, weight, lab values, social history, medical complexities, and surgeries of the patient. The discussion developed and many recommendations were presented for equipment, drug therapies, and referrals to other professionals for more opinions. The patient weighed over 300 pounds at the time of this meeting, but at no time during the meeting was the patient's weight mentioned as a factor in the initiative we were creating.     Could the overweight condition the patient presented be a cause of most of the maladies he or she presented?  If the overweight condition were addressed could the patient return to optimal functioning?   Why were we blinded to the obvious?

There is a saying about "The elephant in the living room". This is what it means. We are blinded by the obvious.

Gwyneth Paltrow is a gorgeous actress.  She is also painfully slim.  For a screen role in the movie "Shallow Hal" she was outfitted in a "fat suit."  I have seen the movie, and I was really struck by her transformation.   Before filming a scene she wore this  'fat suit' at a very expensive hotel often used in movie locations.  She came down in the elevator in her fat suit and walked into the lobby and visited the bar.  In the interview she related how invisible she became.   She was ignored in the bar, and in the elevator she noticed how people looked away.  She attempted to pet some little dogs in the lobby and the owners walked right by her.  For someone accustomed to drawing attention, this was a painful experience.

This is the same phenomenon we see in the treatment rooms of our medical professionals.  If the patient complains of painful feet, a prescription will be written for potent anti-inflammatory drugs even though the obvious cause of these painful feet is a body weighing in excess of 300 pounds.  If an obese patient has high blood pressure and diabetes, prescriptions will be written for these ailments. Perhaps a visit to the diabetic nutritionist will be recommended.   If someone with sleep apnea comes in for treatment, a sleeping monitor will be provided.   The obvious condition may be extreme obesity, but it is not addressed. It is the elephant in the treatment room.

The elephant in the treatment room needs to be examined and understood. Of course we see big. But what made big, big? It is insulin immunity. The visceral fat reservoir created the insulin immunity or insulin resistance. The insulin resistance is the causative factor in obesity and all the related chronic health consequences. When this factor is understood and not feared we can use it to help us heal this difficult syndrome. By reducing the insulin response to the physiology of carbohydrates we can reduce fat mass or lose weight. The improvement to the overall health of the individual will then be coincidental to the reduction of body mass and blood insulin.

How can we meaningfully advise someone who needs help with some of the following?

- Lowering Blood Pressure

- Lowering Blood Sugar

- Relieving Indigestion

- Controlling Irritable Bowel Syndrome

- Lowering Blood Cholesterol, Triglycerides

- Managing Fluid Retention

- Providing Treatment for Sleep Apnea

- Peripheral Neuropathy

- Low back Pain & Foot Pain

# Why You Can't Have Your Cake & Eat It, Too

We need to implement education in the healing of insulin immunity. Our culture is media-driven to consume and to need to consume. Surely we can address this serious health disorder with candor and kindness. We must get beyond the obvious and generate accountability in our social institutions. This accountability must direct the role each of us plays in the creation of health. Accountability on the personal level is the thing that matters when it comes to getting healthy.

Cracking the insulin resistance code is the "coup de grace" in getting a real handle on the cascade of maladies resulting from insulin resistance and glucose toxicity. The number of symptoms you have currently will give us some clues as to how insulin-resistant or sensitive you may be. These signs and symptoms also give us a glimpse at how behaviorally resistant you have become as well.

## Collective Resistance By the Cells

Insulin resistance is the issue. As we have noted, this physiologic phenomenon was first called Metabolic Syndrome X by physician Gerald Reaven, M.D. when he noted an array of conditions appearing as a cluster in his obese patients. These conditions were high blood pressure, NIDDM, coronary artery disease, and abnormal lipids in the blood. As of today, he has expanded this list to include heartburn, gout, and abdominal circumference greater than 30 inches for women and 40 inches for men, fluid retention, and Fibromyalgia. This list will probably increase as we follow more patients. He and others began to see normal-weighted patients showing varying degrees of symptoms, and relating a family history of one or more of the signs listed.  What do all of these people have in common?  The answer is insulin resistance.

It is well known that the abdominal fat mass is very insulin resistant.  This stored body fat sensitizes the body to reject and even repel the hormone insulin.  This rejection could be described as an autoimmune process, for it acts just the same as any allergy.  Once the tissues are demonstrating insulin immunity, insulin resistance usually begins to follow.  It does not go away and often increases  its intensity as one ages.  Even attaining an ideal body weight will not cause insulin resistance to disappear, although it will diminish these responses significantly.  Often hypoglycemic episodes, even reflux will precede and predict the onset of fully involved insulin resistance.

This resistance begins in the vascular systems.  Blood is like an information system, transmitting information much like our information highways work today.  As this liquid transmission travels through the body, it leaves messages within the blood vessel walls.   Lining the veins and arteries are endothelial cells, which transmit command signals responsible for activating the subtle hormonal systems of the body.  This has special significance in our discussions about insulin resistance.  Insulin is produced in the pancreas, which is both an endocrine gland and an exocrine gland.  An endocrine gland releases its hormone directly into the blood supply.  An exocrine gland releases its enzymes directly into the gut.  The enzymes released into the small intestine work on food/fuels such as fat and protein.  The hormone insulin is only activated for one food/fuel type – namely, carbohydrates.

# Why You Can't Have Your Cake & Eat It, Too

It is generally believed that sugar is the substance that binds to insulin. This perception is true; however, it is deceptive. The culprit is actually the product of ALL carbohydrate digestion. This is like the old argument about what comes first, the chicken or the egg. As with carbohydrate consumption, it will become known to your body as one thing, sugar. (Consult the carbohydrate lists in this document for further information on what foods define a carbohydrate.) All carbohydrates yield sugar, even the fat-free, high fiber, natural, organic, fruit, bread, pasta, legumes, and milk products.

Insulin resistance is a definitive process. Exposure to a carbohydrate-rich food/fuel type will stimulate the production of insulin. As soon as carbohydrates are taken into the mouth, the salivary glands begin to communicate to the blood stream that "Sugar is incoming". Insulin production by the pancreas commences. Insulin's only function here is to lower blood sugar. It does this by pushing the sugar into cells. Under "normal" scenarios this will be the end of the game. However, if the individual is genetically insulin-resistant or has acquired insulin resistance, then there is an escalation of events at the cellular level.

Beginning at the cellular walls there is a rejection of insulin and its buddy, glucose. This is now a battle of two gatecrashers, insulin and glucose, as they try to push their way into the theater (the cell) where they are not wanted or needed. The command and control managers in the blood vessel walls (the endothelial cells) are simply doing their job of reporting what is going on in the environment of the blood supply. They will continue to do that regardless of the resistances noted at the cellular level. The endothelial cells will continue to send messages to the pancreas in an effort to contain and control the blood sugar. Because of this intense communication, the pancreas continues to supply insulin in an attempt to reduce the sugar in the blood. Eventually there is a large insulin response/surge to an immovable sugar supply. This is referred to as insulin resistance and glucose toxicity.

This is the dynamic of acquired disorders of our time. There are no exceptions. Culture, race, money, intellect, and will power do not prevent its progress. We are seeing young adults becoming affected earlier with these acquired maladies with alarming speed. Adults are diagnosed with adult-onset diabetes, high blood pressure, high cholesterol, gastro-esophageal reflux, and high triglycerides everyday. We can no longer exclude younger populations from these disorders.

Here is a synopsis of these symptoms and their causes:

## High Blood Pressure or Hypertension

<u>High blood pressure</u> is created by the inability to resolve the high blood sugar and blood insulin levels in the blood supply. The endothelial linings also control dilation and constriction of the vascular tree. With the hyper-insulinemic-glucose-toxic environment, they are unable to perform this function. This is the mechanism responsible for high blood pressure. It is a coincidence how obese individuals have high blood pressure, although some overweight individuals do not. Genetic relationships regulate how insulin insensitivity trickles down into the physiologic pattern. To advance this issue further, weight loss improves blood pressure readings, and blood pressure readings improve with weight management. The perception is correct. The factor improving blood pressure is

the elimination of insulin resistance.  As insulin resistance is reduced, the happy result is lowered blood pressure and weight/fat loss.  The single most significant objective in blood pressure reduction is to reduce the intake of carbohydrate-rich fuels.  This reduces the need for insulin, thereby decreasing the internal stress in the vascular tree.  The blood pressure can then normalize itself and fat can be oxidized.

This miracle can happen within a short period even with less than ten pounds of weight loss.  Blood pressure will stabilize with reduced intake of carbohydrates.  Constant management of carbohydrates will keep your vascular system performing at its best.

**Heartburn or GERD**

<u>Gastro-esophageal reflux disease (GERD)</u> is occurring in epidemic numbers, and is the reason many patients seek treatment.  The complaint is also called heartburn, felt as a backwash of acid high into the esophagus.  Sometimes there is a noticeable hoarseness to the voice.  We know the stomach is a very sensitive hormonal system.  Studies have shown how the stomach depends on the information contained in the blood supply to regulate the speed of emptying.  If the blood sugar is high, then the stomach will hold onto its contents in an effort to control glucose toxicity.  With prolonged elevations in blood sugar, the heartburn or gastro-esophageal reflux will be severe and long lasting.  With repeated exposure to large quantities of carbohydrates when insulin resistance is present, this phenomenon may develop.

This symptom often precedes the evolution of other obesity-related diseases.  The scientific literature has reports of the frequent development of non-insulin-dependent adult-onset diabetes in those previously diagnosed with esophageal reflux disease. GERD is seen in normal-weighted individuals as well. With a careful dietary history one discovers the high intake of carbohydrates. GERD then could be viewed as a warning symptom. It is painful and disruptive, it demands our attention, and most of us cannot ignore it when it appears.

Once I had a patient who came in for diabetes and weight management. What was striking to me was the persistent cough, serious shortness of breath, and hoarseness she displayed. I questioned her about this in the history portion of our session. She related that her practitioner felt this was a bronchospasm and treated her with steroid inhalants. She said it really didn't help, but she took them anyway.

We continued to meet and it became apparent to me that this hoarseness sounded like the stridor one associates with croup in a child. I asked her if she had reflux, and she said she didn't. She said her doctor was monitoring her lungs, but something was not right. We talked and I suggested she needed to visit a specialist who deals with upper airway conditions, an ear, nose, and throat specialist. It took three months for her to get a referral and an authorization from her insurance company.

The specialist scheduled her for an immediate bronchoscopy. She came in to see me about two weeks after that procedure was done, bringing the pictures of her larynx. The opening into her airway was less than 5 millimeters. She was in serious trouble of losing her airway. What also showed on the pictures were small ulcers in the trachea. I asked her what caused these erosions in the airway. She said the specialist told her it was caused by gastric reflux. She was obviously short of breath at the time and I told her I was very concerned about her airway. She related she was not supposed to go out of the house, but she wanted me to see her pictures.

A few weeks later she called me. I could hardly make out who it was on the phone. Then she told me she had had an emergency tracheotomy. After spending eight days in the intensive care unit and a few more days in the hospital, she came home. She said life was not worth living like this, she was crying and so depressed. Gastro-esophageal reflux can be a very dangerous presenting symptom. We may blow it off as simple indigestion, but that would be a big mistake.

We must learn to recognize when the door opens. We are programmed to resist and deny these problems. We may even devalue them. Symptoms are a door opening our awareness to what is present.

It is important to give this symptom the full attention it requires. Medication is helpful but it is not an end in itself. Often I see individuals who take the medication, while doing nothing with adjusting the diet. The medicines used for the treatment of GERD are expensive and usually not covered by insurance. If the insurance company does cover it, it does so at higher co-pay. When these drugs go over-the-counter, then the full cost impact is felt. This symptom is important and costly.

## Irritable Bowel Syndrome

<u>Crohn's Disease or Irritable Bowel Syndrome, Celiac disease</u> is another problem caused by ingesting large quantities of

carbohydrates. It is experienced as a frequent dumping of the contents of the bowel. Often this is as unpleasant as it is unpredictable. This particular problem originates in the small intestine, when large amounts of partially undigested carbohydrates will escape from the small intestine to be dropped into the large bowel. Carbohydrates are very hydrophilic, which means they have an affinity for water. Like a magnetic attraction, a large amount of water is pulled out of the body and floods the large bowel with fluids. The irritant effect of the undigested carbohydrates plus the large amount of body fluid will propel this flood with some force. Often there is cramping, gas, even bleeding. Severity will increase with exposure to the carbohydrate-rich fuels in the diet. Insulin sensitivity may or may not be a factor.

Some patients also relate alternating episodes of constipation with this syndrome. In all, the toll of this unpleasantness is disruption and pain. These problems are very costly in terms of one's ability to enjoy life in the sense of physical economics. Individuals who are willing to attempt the decrease in carbohydrates relate an improvement or elimination of their irritable bowel issue. One patient related to me the immediate return of all of her irritable bowel symptoms with one carbohydrate indiscretion. Her life had been made miserable by the burning, distention, cramping, and loose frequent stools. She related how she had lived with this misery for years. Often taking prescribed medication with no relief, she contemplated a gastrectomy.

In three months time, she had complete relief, so she decided her bowel and stomach must be healed. She told me she had one piece of white cake with frosting, and in a few hours the entire gut was afire. Like any allergy, if we eliminate the allergen we find most of our symptoms are relieved. Then if we are exposed to that substance, the entire syndrome is ignited. When we met for a visit, she told me how she didn't believe me when I had told her that her bad gut was the result of her carbohydrate habit. She also doubted she would ever feel normal again. So when she experienced normal bowel movements, she was impressed. Yet, she needed some more research and development. Experience is a very good teacher.

## High Cholesterol, High Triglycerides

Hyperlipidemia is a complex of increasing cholesterol and triglycerides in the blood. Triglycerides and cholesterol are compounds created by the liver, resulting from the reactivity of high blood sugar and too much blood insulin. The human body does not make cholesterol from eating eggs or peanuts. Cholesterol is triggered by the reaction of an oversupply of insulin to the immovable blood sugar levels. It is the same with triglycerides. Triglycerides are the compounding of glucose particles into a storable form of energy moved into the adipose layer for later use. Often these lipids remain in the blood supply.

In studies done on dogs, this phenomenon was demonstrated. While it pains me to think of animals being used in this way, I was stunned by the findings. In the live experiment, insulin was infused into the femoral artery of dogs. In a short time, the femoral artery became thickened with cholesterol deposits. We have known about this finding for many years, but relating of to the sickness it causes was missed. In the artery, hyperinsulinemia was artificially induced. In humans who consume huge amounts of carbohydrates, they become over time hyper-insulinemic.

Hyper-insulinemia is just a big word for huge amounts of insulin. This huge amount of insulin can be found in circulating blood in those individuals who also have high cholesterol and high triglycerides. High cholesterol has been shown in normal-weighted non-obese insulin-resistant individuals as well as overweight insulin-resistant individuals. Since insulin is a responder to the stimulus of carbohydrates, it behooves us to respect the relationship when we are trying to correct cholesterol and triglycerides.

**Coronary Artery Disease**

<u>Coronary artery disease</u> is another outcome of glucose toxicity and insulin resistance. Think of the blood supply filled with blood sugar levels, loads of insulin, cholesterol, and triglycerides. This becomes like a toxic sludge moving through the cardiovascular system, slowly irritating the endothelial linings and causing inflammation. This is the process responsible for undermining the health of our veins and arteries. Clogging, irritations, and hyper coagulation are caused by glucose toxicity.

**Adult-Onset Diabetes**

<u>Non-Insulin-Dependent Diabetes Mellitus</u> or NIDDM is by now an epidemic in our middle age population. Unfortunately, NIDDM is striking even younger populations. The normal values for fasting blood sugars are 70-110 in this day. Thirty years ago, normal values were 70-100. There are some practitioners who will say a 120 fasting blood sugar is normal,

as a matter of political correctness. Experience has shown that increasing blood sugar levels have corresponded to increasing disease states in humans. Early warning symptoms are excessive thirst, excessive urinary frequency, and extraordinary hunger. There is only one food type that stimulates insulin -- carbohydrate.

When the blood sugar is high and remains elevated, the body reacts by providing insulin to match up with the glucose. Normally the body does this quite well, but there can be a catch. Visceral body fat is insulin-resistant. A family history of any of the foregoing symptoms is a timetable for the development of insulin resistance. Indicators include a large abdominal fat mass, a history of coronary artery disease, high blood pressure, gastro-esophageal reflux, irritable bowel syndrome, and hyper-lipidemia.

## Fluid Retention

The constant feeding and re-feeding, creates the line-crasher story again and again. It is self-compounding and very destructive. Typically this insulin/glucose/cortisol dynamic causes <u>fluid retention</u>. This is a built-in protection mechanism designed to pull fluid around the vital organs. The kidneys, sensing this chaos in the "hallway" of the blood supply, will start holding on to water just in case something bad happens. This is the water released early in low-carbohydrate eating plans. It can be very deceptive, tricking us into believing we are losing fat when we are just releasing stored water. Retained fluid release will occur during the first two to three weeks of low-carbohydrate high-protein dieting.

# Why You Can't Have Your Cake & Eat It, Too

It will take at least three weeks to consistently release fat. When weight is regained quickly after the consumption of a large amount of carbohydrates, it most likely will be fluid. The stress response returns quickly to the body. The first response to sudden high-carbohydrate intake will most certainly be fluid retention.

## High/Low Energy Fluctuations

Back in the line, waiting patiently is stored fat and protein. The body prefers to use its high-octane fat and amino acids, but it cannot. The burly insulin forces the glucose to the head of the line, so the fat can't get going into energy production, even though the body prefers to use its fat. Insulin commands a high price. So in a very interesting way, insulin becomes a signal for the body to hold onto its fat. It is a paradox, but an interesting one. In order for the body to give up its fat, then, insulin production needs to be minimal. Fat is the body's preferred fuel, not sugar -- the stuff of carbohydrates.

This is the big reason portion-control dieting doesn't work. It doesn't work because the individual has signature insulin tolerances. It is important to learn what your insulin sensitivity is. This is the point where the body is perking along burning its high octane fat, weight is being lost, symptoms are diminishing, and those awful highs and lows of energy are gone.

The <u>highs and lows of energy</u> occur as large amounts of insulin finally overtake the cells and move large amounts of glucose into the cell. Returning to our line-crashers idea, once the insulin pushes its buddy's glucose into the cell, the bottom, the energy, drops out. This is an awful feeling of heavy feet and knuckles dragging on the ground. During the time that blood sugar and blood insulin compete within the bloodstream, the immune response within the cells gets fired. This creates a delay in the delivery of energy to the muscle fibers. In the time between the intake of carbohydrates and the resolution of glucose into the cells there is a delay or wait, as I like to call it. It is in this time and space that we have the experience of fatigue in energy levels.

## Chronic Fatigue and Fibromyalgia

Fatigue, sore muscles, and hunger become familiar companions. In another way, this is also the beginning of muscle soreness and the Fibromyalgia complex.

Fibromyalgia is a word referring to pain in the muscles. The "fibro" prefix suggests the muscle has become fibrous. Simply stated, the muscles are not getting nutrients. Remember, when blood sugar is elevated, blood is not getting into the cell. Likewise, fat and protein are not being utilized because of the presence of insulin. This results in a form of starvation to the muscle fibers, which leads to pain and a feeling of being knotted up.

These sore and starving muscle areas can become progressively more painful, which will lead to severe leg pain and pain in other areas. Remember, when the blood sugar remains high, muscle cannot get nutrients. Further complicating this process is the cellular destruction accompanying this malnutrition. Often small areas of muscle become fibrous or knotted. There is unrelenting fatigue with spasmodic pain in the muscles. The connective tissues supporting the muscles become strained and it becomes difficult to ambulate.

This is a form of malnutrition. Many years ago we had epidemics of severe vitamin deficiency, especially Vitamin C, D, and K. We remember how groups of people became seriously ill from the deprivation of these important intrinsic elements. When sailors began to put lime and orange juice into their rations of rum, they noticed the scurvy wasn't so bad. They used these juices for hundreds of years before we knew about the importance of Vitamin C.

We have a long way to go before we can change in our belief systems. Let's hope it is not 250 years.

## Neuropathy and Ulcers

At some point there is change in the type and character of the pain felt in the extremities. Complaints of dullness, numbness, burning, and abrupt pain in the extremities signal the beginning of a term we call peripheral neuropathy. This complication is a signal that tissue destruction is beginning in the extremities. In medical lingo, extremity is the same as peripheral. Most of the time this burning pain is felt in the feet, with painful burning first, then numbness, then ulcers.

The nerves in the starving muscle groups feel this severe pain. In some cases there is vascular impairment to the legs. This impaired circulation results in frequent infections with ulcerations.

We have a saying referring to "Having our legs knocked out from under". Another common saying talks about having "The rug pulled out from under" us. These are interesting phrases, because one of the long-term consequences of out- of-control blood sugar can be the loss of one's feet or toes. Symbolically speaking, this is having the rug pulled out from under us.

On the other side of the painful aspects of this disorder is the complication known as a loss of feeling to the lower extremities, which can result in unintentional injuries to these areas. Because of the impaired circulation, these small injuries can become very significant. There are small injuries done to the blood vessels, nerves and muscles by insulin resistance, which will result in big problems with the legs and feet.

Adequate protein intake, decreased intake of carbohydrates, moderation in fat use, lots of water, and plenty of rest improve these types of muscular pain. The resultant fat loss constitutes a significant improvement as well. Weight is removed from the muscles and joints. Nutrients are being utilized on a regular basis. Cellular resistance is no longer the obstacle that it once was. Food and water are no longing waiting. Nutrition is doing its job. Remember this muscle soreness returns as soon as high-carbohydrate eating is resumed. It does not go away.

## Sleep Apnea and Sleep Disturbances

Earlier in the discussion, this condition was mentioned, but it is important to repeat how disruptive frequent awakenings and urinary frequency are. Often the individual falls asleep during the day at inopportune times, even while driving. Yawning, deep sighing, and napping frequently are seen during the day.

# Why You Can't Have Your Cake & Eat It, Too

This is oxygen starvation. Oxygen is a part of the nourishment of the body. Imagine the chest compressed with stored body fat. Lifting the musculature of the chest containing large amounts of fat is exhausting work. We breathe approximately twenty respirations per minute. During sleep, there are fewer respirations.

The chest is restricted in its capacity to exchange oxygen when there are large stores of fat in the area. The chest muscles work to keep oxygen going into the lungs. Respirations become less frequent during sleep apnea. There are moments when all of this just stops. There is also a fat pad in the back of the throat, which will also compress the breathing space. Snoring followed by silence is the sound of sleep apnea. Some individuals will talk about nightmares jolting him or her awake as a result of apnea.

Urinary frequency is typical of persons with sleep apnea, as the result of the volume overload the heart produces during the time of no breathing. The heart goes into overdrive to get oxygen to the vital areas of the body. This overdrive will produce a type of hormone from the kidneys that will result in the release of the volume overload. This will be experienced as urinary frequency during the night. Some folks go through this cycle as often as every hour throughout the night. It becomes a double-edged sword. One has the lack of sleep and the apnea when they try to sleep.

Sleep apnea is now seen in overweight young adults. Twenty something's who are overweight are having trouble staying asleep and keeping awake. Young adults who are overweight will sometimes have their day-to-night schedules reversed. They will sleep all day, and be up at night. While this might

174

appear to be anti-social in the family dynamic, it may indicate a type of adaptation to the sleep apnea.  The only way they can sleep deeply is to be the exhausted night owl.

Sleep apnea is very hard on the heart.  With chronic long-standing sleep apnea, the heart can go into irregular rhythms which will require medication and treatment by a cardiologist.  Occasionally the heart rhythms will send the patient into treatment, and not the sleep apnea.  The sleep apnea is undiscovered, and therefore not reported or even suspected.

## Chapter Six:
## All-Consuming Passions

### Persistent Resistance

As the fuel mix of nutrients is corrected to match the individual variables of insulin resistance, weight is lost and symptoms dissipate. Progress toward an ideal body size and improvements in health are noted. Often it is at this point that relapses in eating behaviors are seen. Another way to look at it is as a type of "Research and development" which produces immediate physiologic meltdown. Some will say they didn't realize how miserable they felt when they ate loads of carbohydrates all the time. Others will talk about how good they felt while on the high protein, low-carbohydrate program. Yet, they relapsed.

Relapses are good learning experiences. They teach many lessons. One of these is how freely we take our health for granted. One day we are taking our high blood pressure for granted. Then in a couple of weeks, the high blood pressure is normal. It may stay that way for months. Then we test the waters by increasing the intake of carbohydrate-rich foods. We react with surprise at how quickly the high blood pressure symptom returns. We are astonished with the swift return of fluid retention, indigestion, even the energy fluctuations. The speed of symptom return is dizzying. Seemingly, getting rid of these problems took forever. Now they are back. Is this regression?

This unpleasant consequence demonstrates the progression of insulin resistance. One might think insulin resistance can be arrested when a corrected eating style is implemented. A

corrected eating style will suspend the insulin resistance for the time being. Should old eating styles be resumed, the insulin resistance takes off right where it was last active.
Usually the progress of time enhances the severity of insulin resistance. What one could tolerate in terms of carbohydrates will be much less, day-by-day and year-by-year. Fine wine is the only thing that improves with age.

Carbohydrate intolerance may intensify at interesting times in one's life. Pregnancy and menopause seem to be events when glucose intolerance and insulin resistance overlap. Retirement may parallel this phenomenon, and there may be other circumstances which will create this kind of parallel. But often the "event" gets the attention rather than the physical symptoms. "This caused that" or 'That caused this." The explanations are varied. The fact is, insulin resistance and glucose toxicity can be genetic, environmental, and time dependent. A circumstance may have nothing to do with insulin resistance and its appearance. The circumstance may help you remember when these things started to change. Physical disease gets the attention, and our conflicted life circumstances are discounted.

## My Story

We become the disease rather than experiencing it as something that needs our attention. A long time ago, doctors were referred to as "attending' physicians." They were giving attention to the patient in an effort to help him through his moments of illness. Disease is really being not at ease. What has happened in our moments of ease to cause us to be ill? What needs attending to?

# Why You Can't Have Your Cake & Eat It, Too

A few years ago, I experienced a retinal detachment, which created a disturbance in my vision.  It was a sudden shock to my sensory system, threatening my ability to see clearly.  A brown curtain was being lowered in my eye.  It was terrifying.  It required swift medical and surgical intervention.  My physician referred me as an emergency to an eye specialist.  I went immediately to the office and waited about three hours to be seen.  After the exam the doctor told me it was too late to help me, I was going to lose my sight.  I was devastated.  He said he would notify my doctor.  The door was left open as he made the call; I noticed how quickly he returned to the exam room.  He told me my doctor wanted another opinion from a retinal surgeon.  The office was calling for me and I should leave immediately to go to see him.

My husband was now enlisted as my chauffeur, for my vision was limited.  Soon I was in a waiting room full of people who had had eye surgery.  I looked at them; they looked at me.  It would seem that they could see me better than I could see myself.  After the surgeon examined the eye, he said we needed to go to surgery as soon as possible.  There was still time to save my eye.  There was grace, and it was being extended to me.  As I waited to get information about the surgery, a fellow patient came to me and said, "Try not to worry. You will be okay.  I will pray for you."  There was a moment of more grace.

The surgery was completed and I went to recover my sight.  I was flat on my stomach for 3 weeks in order to hold in position the gas bubble that was being used to splint the retina in place.  I have had three more surgeries since that time, and now see 20/30 in that eye.  It is a miracle of science, math, effort, and opportunity all meeting in the same moment for me.

## Why You Can't Have Your Cake & Eat It, Too

The journey could have been very different if I had chosen to believe my situation was hopeless.

During the time of my recovery, I had time to contemplate the meaning of this experience. I was in the process of regaining my vision and my health. I wanted to explore the incident that had come my way. As an emerging healing professional, I knew that on some level I needed a look at the entire picture. I promised myself, and the Universe, that I would not avoid any unpleasant messages that came to me during this time of self-examination. This would become another chapter in the book of revelations. After all, I was offered the opportunity to restore my sight. I didn't want to miss anything.

I asked myself a series of questions. What had I lost sight of? What did I need to see? What did I not want to see? What had happened to my vision? What would I do with the new vision when I got it? I had to acknowledge my attachment to my work. Not only did I work in a medical practice, but I was also working toward developing my intuition for use in the clinical area. My time off work for regaining my vision was the purpose. I needed the time to regain my vision.

My vision did change, and expand. I chose to take the opportunity I had to establish a wellness-coaching business. This practice would incorporate all dimensions of healing human nutritional needs. In a few short months I was starting to see clients/patients. A part of this vision would be writing all the information I had gathered about human nutrition into a workbook. Then I completed my training as a practitioner of insight and intuition. I could see hunger for connection, knowledge, and direction as a valuable part of nurturing the human spirit to choose life-enhancing behaviors. I saw the inside of the patient being reflected on the outside.

So I contemplated how I see the earth and humanity through the lens of what Thich Nhat Hanh calls inter-being. I had to acknowledge the many plant and animal species that are becoming extinct due to the rapid expansion of human populations. I had to acknowledge how resources such as energy and water, once thought to be endless, were becoming scarce. This scarcity was brought about by the insatiable demand of people for water, land, and energy. This meant that some of us had it all, and some of us had nothing. The balance of power was switched to the disrupters. Indeed, we are experiencing power outages all over the world. We have become tangled rather than inter-related.

As I applied this information to the problem of obesity, I could see some interesting parallels. The expanding waistlines represent the expansions of human populations. As our populations change locations, large pieces of nature are converted into parking lots. What was flexible has now become rigid. Animals and plants are relocated if they survive the influx of humanity. Some animals are turned into road kill. Sometimes animals are unable to adjust and find their way into urban areas, where they are killed. Water, land, and energy are limited. As humans, our internal life-sustainers are limited as well. Yet we push ourselves as we push the environment for more of everything. As we consume the earth, we consume ourselves. The resources we take for granted, both internally and externally, are finite.

## Why You Can't Have Your Cake & Eat It, Too

When our community's hospital was first built, it was located on a large parcel of farmland, much of it undeveloped until recently. Along the drive into the hospital complex there lived a community of jackrabbits. They would sit in the shade of the few trees, and we watched them with pleasure year after year. The area was undergoing growth, and after many years, the hospital expanded in size. This included an increase in parking lots, encroaching on the jackrabbit's habitat. A token fenced area was designated for the jackrabbits, as if they could be contained behind a wrought iron fence!

Those of us who observed the changes in this area grimly accepted the fact that the jackrabbits would become road kill. One day I was in one of the high-rise buildings on hospital property overlooking the freeway and the canal. The canal was dry for its yearly maintenance by the city. There in the canal was one lone jackrabbit moving as fast as the traffic in the freeway next to it. That was the last time we saw one. While some might consider a jackrabbit a pest, it is a creature that has adapted to the harsh Sonoran desert. Still it could not adjust to the advancing urban growth.

The sustaining of life as we know it is undergoing change. During such a period, sustaining the conditions necessary for the support of the systems we inhabit is our responsibility. The lowly urban jackrabbit is gone, but not without a cost to the environment. The physical body will need to have internal conditions in place to support it while it changes with age. That too is a part of our responsibility.

The life you have will change. The choices you make will impact those changes. Resisting those choices will create pain.

# Why You Can't Have Your Cake & Eat It, Too

## Making the Best of It

Believe it or not, this is a type of intellectual resistance. Making the best of a situation has the appearance of taking the high moral ground. It is just the opposite. It is putting another person, place, or thing in charge of your best interest. We all know what the word "assume" means. It is true here as well. In making the best of something, we often do it with less than a best effort. How do we create out best effort? How do we create our best intention? It takes practice. Trial-and-error is a formidable teacher. Let us hope we will stay conscious during our experience. Holding on to our center while experiencing meltdown at warp speed will teach us how strong we are.

Sometimes, it is true, we fear succeeding. We will create drama and sabotage to deflect the pain of giving up what we really want or what we truly feel. Deep inside we know this, yet we do it anyway. We tell ourselves that in making the best of something, it will be necessary to postpone doing something else, perhaps a task that had a high priority. But we say, "I was making the best of it". It is as if we have a ready form of justification. Making the best of something may cause us to split off from our intended purpose. We feel deep in our gut there a loss of balance, perhaps even anxiety. Driven by a sense of duty to create the best, or doing it for the best, we are not being true to our purpose. It is a compromise of our goals.

What is worse, this making the "best of it" makes us angry. We wanted to do something a certain way and in a particular time, yet we negotiated our choices and created a postponement or delay. Yes, it became wait and weight.

# Why You Can't Have Your Cake & Eat It, Too

Why? It generated a justification.  Justifications give way to excuse-making, the final touch to "making the best of it."  We pretend we are happy with the postponement, when we really are seething with impatience.  We pretend we are content waiting, when we were really ready to go now.

 At this point, looking at one's intention can be important. Mother Theresa said, "We can do small things with love". The intention of love softens the edges of the heart.  The intention of fear hardens the edges of the heart.

"Making the best of it" is a negative behavior.  It is trading off one type of fiction for another.  The effect on the effort to get healthy means it gets postponed when we are "making the best of things".  Oh yes, this is a very common occurrence. To recover from insulin resistance and glucose intolerance, you must keep your highest intention at work on this journey. Aligning your purpose, your intention, and your actions is the way up and out.  Ask yourself, when poised over your choices, "Does this nourish my soul?"

There will be many erroneous belief systems at work in your emotional and intellectual body, and they can propel you into behavior patterns that are very resistant to change. Resistant on the outside means resistance on the inside.  The patterns of the past, old invalid belief systems, and reactionary behaviors will come back for frequent visits.  Just like unwelcome disturbances, these patterns will sidetrack you into the familiar resistant eating dramas.  It will be important to review your development and your research.  These opportunities demonstrate how much you have improved, and where you need to challenge the old ways of being.

# Why You Can't Have Your Cake & Eat It, Too

We are working on a specific technique for addressing change in nutrition. Overeating, bingeing, sneaky eating, and medicating with food are examples of emotional resistance. Cleaning your plate, the food pyramid, ADA food rules, and portion control are some examples of intellectual resistance. More examples of nutritional resistance exist and are founded on myth. Addressing the internal argument before the event takes place gives us the opportunity to look at things with fresh perspectives.

## Your Ideal Body Weight

Let us presume that you are at your ideal body weight. Your next opportunity is to discover what your nutrient requirements are. Using the assessment forms, make a list of what you currently consume. From that list, create your totals on the concepts you have learned about insulin resistance and nutrient requirements of the human body. Factor in any of the signs or symptoms you may now be experiencing. These signs and symptoms will give you clues as to your emerging insulin resistances. In most cases, your protein intake will need to come up to minimal daily levels. Your carbohydrate intake will need to be reduced to your maximal levels. Inventory your water intake, and begin to increase its use.

Carbohydrates will be the brake or the accelerator in your wellness effort. The more carbohydrates consumed, the slower the progress toward wellness and ideal body size. Lessening one's carbohydrate intake will speed you to your desired wellness and ideal body size. In all cases, protein will need to be consumed every day in keeping with your particular situation.

# Why You Can't Have Your Cake & Eat It, Too

Once you have attained your ideal body weight, you will need to continue to consume protein at the levels required to support this weight.  The only thing to be adjusted will be the carbohydrate intake.  It is most important to go slowly in adding carbohydrates back in.  Doing this  in large amounts is one of the biggest mistakes made in weight control efforts.

For example, suppose your intake of carbohydrates was 50 grams during the time of your wellness plan.

- Once you are at your ideal weight, where you no longer wish to lose more weight,  slowly increase your carbohydrates by 10 grams per week.  To be clear, the first week or two of your weight maintenance your daily carbohydrate intake will be 50 grams.

- Some people will find it advisable to keep the carbohydrate level intake at the reduction level for five days a week, with the addition of 10 grams of carbohydrate two days a week.

- In the third and fourth week of your weight maintenance,  increase your carbohydrates to 70 grams only twice a week.

- Continue at the reduction carbohydrate ceiling the other 5 days.  Make note of how your weight is maintaining.

- If your weight begins to increase at any of the changes made during the first month, then reduce your carbohydrates.

# Why You Can't Have Your Cake & Eat It, Too

- If symptoms such as reflux or fluid retention return, then decrease your carbohydrates.

- Always drink lots of water and continue with the protein.

- A sudden regain of 5 pounds needs to be addressed immediately.

Returning to your old dietary ways will quickly result in rapid weight gain.  It is a very predictable consequence.  Insulin resistance and glucose toxicity remain in the cellular memory.  Once reactivated with high carbohydrate consumption, weight will be regained.  Symptoms will return.

Someone once said that doing the same thing the same way and expecting different results was the definition of insanity.  Try to maintain your weight with the principles you have learned.  Get back on your diet, should you go off course, as quickly as possible.  Don't weight/wait!

Learn to recognize when the door opens.  A door represents a stop or a type of threshold, and also symbolizes resistance.  It is important to welcome doors instead of avoiding them.  You are being given the keys to those doors by way of the techniques you are learning.  When opportunity knocks, as in the old saying, open the door.  Don't shut it.  That is resistance.

## Chapter Seven:
## Getting to Purpose

### Alignments

Here are some helpful tools to use in construction of a dietary recovery process.   Use them to help you form your plan:

- Plug into the written menus some of the items you prefer to eat.

- Remember to implement your nutritional needs according to the formulas you have learned.

- Make copies of the dietary diary to help you with food intake and food values.

- With regard to some recipes or menus you currently enjoy, use the guides to help make them over to fit your current circumstances.

- The statistics you are creating will guide you as your weight changes, blood sugar improves, and blood lipids lower, and other symptoms improve.

- Note your weight on your calendar, updating it weekly.   Sometimes a pattern emerges.   This pattern may help to sustain you when you are waiting for a specific outcome.

This is a purposeful effort.   Your purpose in your diet will emerge each day.  Looking at your day, your routine eating process can include the preparation time needed to put it into action. Washing and cleaning vegetables is a good way to have an added back-up when hunger strikes expectedly. Notice, the word expectedly is used. We can expect to get hungry, so it is important to have a planned-out strategy that fits your lifestyle, all ready to go. Having 4 ounce Baggies of meat ready in the meat drawer or having some kind of high-protein drink available makes your plan fool proof.

Preparation with a purpose will make your plan run smoothly.

## Erroneous Belief Systems

Here is a list of some common beliefs or myths about human nutrition and health:

- Calories-in must equal calories-out

- Dietary protein is destructive to the kidneys

- Sugar is white stuff in the sugar bowl

- Portion control equals weight control

- Exercise to lose weight

- Liquid diets promote faster weight loss

- Muscle weighs more than fat

- Sensible diets work

- Cutting back, pushing back, will promote weight control

# Why You Can't Have Your Cake & Eat It, Too

- Willpower is all you need

- Menopause makes you gain weight

- Speeding up metabolism will produce weight loss

- The diet must be "balanced"

- Sugar-free is good for me

- Protein diets cost more

- You got to have fiber!!!

- This is healthy fat, that is bad fat

- Eggs and nuts give you cholesterol

- Honey is better than sugar

- (Add others here)

# Why You Can't Have Your Cake & Eat It, Too

These perceptions add wait/weight to your effort to succeed at making progress and maintaining the progress you have made. They represent little pockets of resistance, which act like brakes. It may seem as though just as you get started and are moving along, even making progress, then out of "know-where" you bump into one of these perceptions. This 'know-where' may represent some inside-to-outside influence. A belief system from the outside becomes integrated to the inside.

These perceptions come out of your history, present, and awareness. They are then applied like speed bumps on a walk to hobble or sabotage your journey to wellness. Most importantly, none of them are true. They are clever marketing strategies at their worst. At their best, they are meant to explain your health mysteries, but are simply explanations with no basis in fact or science. Each one of us has a particular way to interpret our mysteries. Some of these interpretations can be factual. Some are not.

The following paragraphs are meant to dispel some of your health- or weight-related myths. The frequently repeated myths are drummed into our collective thoughts. Our social groups and families have their mythologies, which are intended to explain why things happen as they do. This is extraordinarily true in the realm of health and wellness.

<u>Counting calories</u> is one of the first things mentioned in weight- management. Usually someone sets a target for your maximum allowed calories per day. You may read something in a magazine that gives you a "set point". You may set an imaginary number of allowed calories based on the

190

# Why You Can't Have Your Cake & Eat It, Too

recommended daily allowances.  There are various ways to arrive at these arbitrary caloric allotments.

The human mind can be a very scary place when it sets out to count calories.  All kinds of gimmickry have been created around counting calories.  There are the non-impact calories.  There are the invisible calories.  I have yet to see someone lose weight on 1,000 calories of M&M's!!  Yet I see this kind of thinking drive the perception about calorie counting.

When someone sets out to achieve energy balances in a diet, an exercise routine is often included.  This is a set-up for disappointment.  The only reason we are taking this path is the expectation that  diet and exercise will provide weight loss.  Living in the expectation that a set amount of exercise plus a set amount of calories will produce weight loss we often experience a poor result. We just don't lose the weight because we are still eating huge amounts of carbohydrates.

The unacknowledged factor in weight management is the hormone insulin.  Insulin is required for  the metabolism of carbohydrate. Because all carbohydrates become sugar, they generate an insulin response.  The presence of insulin disables the body's ability to burn fat.

In a case of misplaced zeal, the sugar cane industry took the hit for the obesity epidemic.  The reality is that all carbohydrates are responsible for the obesity epidemic.  This is true of honey and fructose, as well as pasta, breads, cereals, rice, and legumes. They are all sugar, and whether they are complex or simple is of no consequence.  Carbohydrates become sugar once they are exposed to human digestion.  This sugar will evoke an insulin response.

# Why You Can't Have Your Cake & Eat It, Too

Insulin will then control the rate of fat storage or fat oxidation. A lower volume of blood insulin allows stored fat to be used as energy. Higher levels of blood insulin will promote fat storage.

This high blood insulin responds to high blood carbohydrate/sugar levels in the dietary intake. If we want the blood sugar to come down, we have to eliminate carbohydrates. If we want the blood sugar to come down, we have to eliminate dietary sugars. If we want the blood sugar to come down, then we have to toss out most of the food pyramid.

These insulin levels react to sugar/carbohydrate. Activity from exercise will create a moment of increased insulin-sensitivity to the cells. This activity will endure for the length of time one exercises, and then it is gone. The human body is a fat-burning machine, set up to burn fat as a preferred high-octane fuel. Fat storage is replaced and oxidized every day, if we reduce the need for blood insulin. The only way to do this is to decrease all carbohydrates.

Decreasing carbohydrates does not mean eliminating them. It means learning what you are able to tolerate. Once your tolerances are known, then creating a dietary parallel is all it takes. This may not be politically correct, but carbohydrates must be limited each day. Even the fat-free mentality promotes unlimited sugar/carbohydrate consumption. Those fat-free blueberry muffins are loaded with insulin-inducing carbohydrates. Ditto for the fat-free bialy.

Ask yourself if <u>counting calories</u> has worked for you. Has <u>exercise</u> matched your expectation of weight control? A pound of stored fat represents 3,500 calories. A mile of

# Why You Can't Have Your Cake & Eat It, Too

walking or running expends 110 calories. This means one would have to walk or run 30 miles in one day to burn up one pound of stored body fat. This could take as much as 10 hours. If you are attempting to bicycle away fat, then four miles of bike riding will equal one mile of walking or running.

Protein diets have been vilified by just about everybody, even health professionals. This negative bias against increasing dietary protein is based on the collective thought that says dietary protein is responsible for kidney destruction. Earlier in this writing this was described. Collective thought also has a myth that reflects a bias against red meat. This goes to the belief that red meat promotes cholesterol production. This is simply not true. Glucose in the blood initiates insulin. Individual reactions to insulin may promote cholesterol imbalances as a part of the toxic phenomenon. This was demonstrated a long time ago on studies with dogs and recently with humans.

Protein diets are often described as "expensive". This may be true in terms of time involved to plan and prepare protein. Protein also said to "cost" a lot of money. Your time and money are the very reason this type of diet is helpful to you. Your health and well-being are priceless. Trips to your doctors, co-pays, time off work, time out of life, and expanding wardrobes are expensive, too.

Does muscle weigh more than fat? Does a pound of muscle weigh more than a pound of fat? A pound is a pound, no matter what that pound is. It takes two pounds of muscle to carry fifty pounds of fat. So if you lose 50 pounds of weight, you will not need two pounds of muscle. So, it is a very interesting compromise. Remember, a pound is a pound. A pound of feathers will take up more space than a pound of steel. But, they will both weigh one pound. Try to remember how much work is involved in building fat from exercise. In women it can take as long as six months of daily work to build just a small amount of muscle. Men will build muscle a little bit faster, but it will far below the expected result. We just don't have the time to devote to 8-hour work-out days. An interesting statistic is 10 pounds of muscle requires only 75 calories of energy.

What, after all, is a <u>balanced diet</u>? What is a <u>sensible diet</u>? The answer to those questions resides in the collective mind which will dictate the balance and sensibility. Usually families, working groups, and the media have the most impact on the perceptions of balance and sensibility. Balanced and sensible eating will reflect the food pyramid in most situations. Then the family will have several food rituals that will dictate what foods will be eaten when. The media adds its spin to the cultural messages. The food pyramid ideology is the framework or the backdrop for these concepts. The ideal of <u>healthy eating</u> usually means eating the food pyramid. The food pyramid contains 500-600 grams of carbohydrate and very little micronutrient. While the perception of the food pyramid is wholesome, and full of nutrition, the reality is different.

The food pyramid was a political and economic solution for food distribution. The FDA had no scientific basis for this food plan. When I ask my clients to explain how the food pyramid came into existence, they relate that it came into being because of the best research and development the United States Government could provide. The reality was and is that the special interest groups built the food pyramid. There is no science today or in history that supports the human nutritional need for all of the items on the food pyramid. The food pyramid represents a piece of the economic pie that excludes the public health and protects the special interests. The food pyramid with its high carbohydrates, low protein, and low fat belief system is directly responsible for the epidemic of obesity today.

## Chapter Eight:
## Reformatting and Reforming

### Reading Labels

Lately, label reading and label writing have become both popular and creative. Some of the labels I have read will swear that a given food item contains 2.9 grams of carbohydrates and is fat-free, with a calorie total on the label of perhaps 100. So where is the truth here? 2.9 grams of carbohydrates would be less than 12 calories. That leaves 88 calories unaccounted for. Even with my limited math skills, I know that doesn't add up.

Trusting label writers is probably not a good idea. Get a nutrition book that will act like a food dictionary. Read up on the foods you frequently use. Protein has 4 calories in a gram. Carbohydrates have 4 calories in a gram. Fat has 9 calories in a gram. Do the math. Do the calories add up?

Recently a new category of carbohydrates has appeared, called non-impact carbohydrates. On the product label are instructions to subtract this non-impact carbohydrate value from the total number of carbohydrates in that item. The same instruction is also seen with the carbohydrate entity known as fiber. This type of labeling is intentionally misleading. Fiber does become sugar. Non-impact carbohydrates are also known as "sugar alcohol", and they too become sugar. My work with diabetics, along with some of the latest research clearly indicate that these new classifications of carbohydrates do cause blood sugar elevations.

196

## Why You Can't Have Your Cake & Eat It, Too

Another clever classification for carbohydrates has been "the glycemic index." The intention with this type of labeling was to measure the anticipated blood sugar response from a particular type of food. The more refined the food, the faster the blood sugar responded. The glycemic index of a food was thought to measure two things: the amount of sugar in the item, and the speed at which the blood sugar became elevated. The glycemic food index then could be used as a guide to direct one's safe use of carbohydrates. The big problem with the glycemic index is its basic assumption that all foods will react the same way in all individuals. We know that each of us is different. <u>We are individual</u>. We will all react differently to food, aspirin, alcohol, and milk products, for example. Once one becomes insulin-resistant, the glycemic index protocols will not work. If one then goes on to become diabetic, the glycemic index is worthless. The insulin-resistant and the diabetic will demonstrate extreme elevations to the blood sugar without regard for its glycemic rating.

Glycemic index, like non-impact carbohydrates, is another creative way to manage the marketing of these types of foods. Dietitians are unable to agree about these classifications. The consumer is easily convinced when a professional organization endorses a particular theory. Some very credible authorities, even Dr. Atkins, have protein bars made with sugar alcohol.

Let's get to the bottom line. Sugar alcohol, fiber, and glycemic foods are carbohydrates. All carbohydrates become blood sugar. Raising blood sugar will create a compensatory insulin release. Each one of you has a particular level of glucose toxicity and insulin resistance. Remember we are uniquely individual.

# Why You Can't Have Your Cake & Eat It, Too

A good place to start evaluating your level of insulin resistance and glucose toxicity is to eliminate carbohydrates for seven days.  Be sure you eat your protein, drink water, and take your vitamins.    Then slowly add in ten grams of carbohydrate a day.   Stay at this 10-gram limit for one week.  Build in additional 10-gram increments in carbohydrates each week.   See how you do.    Note the reappearance of indigestion, irritable bowel, fluid retention, and cravings.  Also note the by-product of your lowered carbohydrate-intake: weight loss.  This weight loss will give you clues as to your insulin sensitivity and glucose intolerance.    The more carbohydrates added to the diet, the slower the weight loss will be.  It is helpful to note this on a calendar or journal.

## Do the Math

We can do the calculations to determine the levels of nutrient intake, using the formula presented here as a beginning in this determination.  If  weight loss is slow or not progressing at all, then the carbohydrate portion of the calculation will have to be revised downward.

First you will have to decide on what your particular Ideal body weight should be.  This  should represent a combination of your lean body mass with an appropriate amount of residual fat mass, somewhere between 10% for males or 25% for females.  Most importantly, each person will determine what is comfortable and sustainable for him or her.

We calculate dietary intake based on the protein requirement for the individual.   Protein intake is determined from the kilogram weight.  To obtain the kilogram weight, just divide the Ideal body weight by 2.2.   Once this value is determined, multiply it by 1.5 Grams of protein.  This will be the minimal amount of protein to be consumed in the diet.

Another way to determine the protein need is to allow one ounce of protein per each ten pounds of Ideal body weight. For example, if the desired weight is 150 pounds, then the protein need will be 15 ounces.  After the protein intake has been determined, the maximum carbohydrate intake should be 50 grams or less.  Depending on many of the physiologic factors we have discussed, the carbohydrate intake may be adjusted up or down.   In some cases 36 grams of carbohydrates may be excessive. The fat intake should be the same as the carbohydrate intake.  The fat will be from added fat, such as oil, mayonnaise, and butter, not the existing fat in food.  .

The ratio of intake will be roughly  2 to 1 to 1.  That is,  protein will have a value of 2,  carbohydrate will have the value of 1 and so will the fat.  It is important to keep these ratios clean, as a food intake plan that is 1 to 1 will not be as productive as the 2 to 1.  What matters most is your own personal choice and comfort level.  This eating strategy does not count calories although one will find the eating plan will contain somewhere between 1000 to 1400 calories.  The fat reserves on your body will make a significant contribution to your energy requirements.

**This is a different way of looking at portion control and calorie counting.  It does measure portions  and calories, but  just not the way we are used to thinking of them.**

# Why You Can't Have Your Cake & Eat It, Too

## Let's Talk Turkey About Pizza

Pizza is one of the most destructive fast foods known to the human race. It raises blood sugar and blood insulin for a longer time than a similarly constructed meal. This can be a negative result for someone trying to control weight, blood sugar, blood insulin, and cravings. Why this is so is still being researched. In the "for what it is worth" column, stay away from pizza. Drive around the block if you have to.

Many will tell you how tempting pizza is. It is eaten in the office, at home, and in the car. It is even good cold. As beguiling as pizza is, it was noted to derail blood sugar management in diabetics. Professional nutritionists noted that pizza-eating diabetics had difficulty in getting blood sugar in compliance. In the one study done, blood sugar and blood insulin stayed high for as long as 15 hours after a meal of two pieces of pepperoni pizza. And if the blood sugar remained elevated, then the blood insulin was elevated as well.

The research could not account for this prolonged elevation, but it noted that more research had to be done. The comparison meal was a turkey sandwich on white bread with mayonnaise and cheese. Six hours after eating this, blood sugar and blood insulin in the comparison meal had begun to decline.

This is a very significant consequence for a nutritional strategy. Consequences of returning to a high carbohydrate eating style are felt immediately. Individual sensitivities to the effects of insulin can have the impact of a stun gun. Glucose toxicities manifest with magnum force. It can take days or even weeks to return to the former state of nutritional compliance. Each person will feel immediately the effects of going on and off his diet.

In some circles there is an interesting collective belief regarding taking certain liberties with the regimen, centered on the idea of eating whatever you want for one day a week. An extreme level of this type of belief would be eating whatever you want for one meal a day, and I have seen this carried out. In either example, this type of an eating strategy will be very discouraging. It is an erroneous belief based on some ill-conceived idea of rewards. The intention is to reward oneself with food for the experience of deprivation.

Almost immediately, the body feels the high levels of blood sugar and blood insulin. Fluid retention and indigestion return. Fat oxidation stops immediately as the body switches onto sugar-rich fuels. Abruptly the body is put into reverse. This momentary inertia will be short-lived. Soon endothelial dysfunction returns, and the cycle of insulin resistance is also in place. This constellation of effects can remain in the metabolism for seven to ten days at its worst. Some people relate feeling the effects of sugar-induced coma for two weeks.

Some commercial diets will tell you that three days should be the extent of your indiscretions. Should you continue to be inappropriate with food one day each week or one meal each day? The mathematical progression of effect will accumulate in wait and weight. Yes, layers of time and work will be require to return to your wellness routine.

Another problem is the amount of time one spends mentally, figuring out how to repair the damage. The damage hardest to repair is related to the amount of time you have to spend on living in your head.  Adding and subtracting all day long can be exhausting.  It is much easier to just "do it."  Telling lies is exhausting.  How do you remember which one to believe?  You know the ones.  Aren't sizes smaller these days?

Having serious health-related illness associated directly to glucose toxicity is a form of deprivation.  Is it not?  Reflux?  Irritable bowel?  High-blood pressure?  Diabetes?  Sleep apnea? Weight gain?   The list goes on from there.  Surely, these things deprive the individual of a fully-involved life.  They rob society of productive individuals.

This loss of usefulness is felt on many levels -- in the family, society, and in the workplace.  Our great society is on the brink of a serious epidemic.  Over half of our adults have obesity.  One third of young people are obese.  There are more non-insulin-dependent diabetics diagnosed now than ever before. For the first time in many years, our longevity statistics are being adjusted downward.  This is true with youngsters as well.  The health consequences of this type of an epidemic will cripple our health care systems.  Economically, the workplace will lose effectiveness.  The family will labor to provide care for afflicted family members.  Industry will shift more cost of health care onto the consumer as well as society.  Our inter-relatedness, and inter-being is going to be tested.

If two thirds of a nation were at risk of an epidemic wouldn't someone raise the alarm?  TB, AIDS, even polio don't have this broad base of victims.  We have in our hands the responsibility for the cause and the cure of this epidemic.  Therefore, choose well. This is metabolic brinkmanship.

## Why You Can't Have Your Cake & Eat It, Too

### Undernourished and Overfed

This would seem to be a paradox.  How could one be overfed yet undernourished?  How could one be malnourished and not hungry?  How could there be children sent to school under-nourished?  How could our senior citizens have malnutrition?  The occurrence of malnutrition from lack of food is much less frequent than the occurrence of malnutrition from being over-fed.  Said another way, more people are overfed and are mal-nourished than are underfed and malnourished.

Going to school with a breakfast of cereal, banana, and milk?  This is a meal of pure sugar.   Bagel and fruit is another typical meal plan.  Most people, or children, run out of "gas" or energy within two or three hours as the blood sugar drops.  This simple blood sugar drop may account for the lack of concentration and disturbances in learning in the classroom.  The next meal arrives from the vending machine or in the lunch line, and it is typically fat-free and high-carbohydrate.  The cycle is repeated many times during the day and for years to come.   The typical lifelong diet is woefully deficient in protein, fat, and water.

Another nutrient-delinquent diet is the frozen or canned convenience-type foods.  This class of foods is labeled with wholesome names and reliable colors.  The fact is that these foods are sugar-water with food color. A minute amount of protein is lumped into a congealed form that liquefies when heated.  It becomes a certainty that we see states of inability to concentrate, confusion, even depression that may be corrected with proper nutrition.  Malnutrition is serious and needs to be corrected with appropriate protein, carbohydrates, fat, and water.

# Why You Can't Have Your Cake & Eat It, Too

**Humanity is in danger of depleting itself at all levels of the life spectrum**.

The American industrialized culture has been indoctrinated into the high-carbohydrate, low-fat eating plan for years.  As a country, we drink more sugar-laden soda pop than water. Generations of families continue this type of nutrition.  An interesting trend is developing, of being undernourished and dehydrated.  Protein is feared, because It is believed to raise cholesterol and cause kidney failure.  People lose their health and their hair, and have frequent episodes of confusion combined with fatigue.  Yet they cannot connect these important dots.  We are busy saving the whales, but we waste the water.  Water is fluid energy.  Its use in hydrating our bodies is underestimated.  Chronic dehydration is a serious health risk.  Chronic malnutrition is going to consume us.

Hundreds of years ago, we had a nutritional disease known as scurvy. This disease would cause bleeding gums and sores on the skin that would not heal.  By a stroke of pure luck someone drew the connection between eating citrus fruit, the improvement of the bleeding gums, and the healing of the sores to the body.  It would take two hundred years for ascorbic acid to be identified. Humans continued to use citrus fruits as a cure for  scurvy before we understood the science.

The high-carbohydrate low-fat low-protein culture has created a plague.  While it may be difficult to see someone who is very overweight as starving, this is really what is taking place.

# Why You Can't Have Your Cake & Eat It, Too

## Food Reformation

Reformers are often severely criticized for their vision. Martin Luther and Martin Luther King were reformers. One was attempting to reform the church of his time. The other was attempting to reform the social order of his time. History gives us a vivid picture in words describing the struggles these two reformers endured. Martin Luther King was murdered for his belief in equal opportunity. Martin Luther was banished from his community. We identify the changes brought about by these reformers with their names.

A short time ago, in 1965 to be precise, I was a student nurse going through my maternity nursing rotation. It was really a long time ago,. Being a part of the delivery room team was an awe-inspiring experience for me, full of moments of suspense interspersed with joy. In the hours of laboring there could be moments of hope. One of the tools I learned was the importance of being positive, appreciative, and supporting of the evolving mothers. I saw how much they needed to be encouraged for the progress they were making, and how much this cheerleading nurtured them. Funny thing, it nurtured me, too.

But I digress. Our fearless maternity-nursing instructor gave us an assignment one time, to read a book called, "Dear Dr. Semelweiss." Most medical professionals will have an instant recognition when this important medical man's name is mentioned. Dr. Semelweiss instituted the simple reform of hand washing between patients.

During his time, there was a terrible epidemic of childbed fever, which usually ended the life of the mother. Sometimes the infant survived, but often the child succumbed as well. Laboring women, who gave birth at home, seemed to do well, and so did their babies, whereas the women who were attended by the physicians of the day in the 1800's developed terrible post-partum infections and died as a result. Women who gave birth in the hospitals of the day also became gravely ill and died. It became a virtual death sentence to give birth in an institution, attended by a doctor. The women of these times knew that to give birth in the hospitals would mean certain death, so many of them had unattended births, at home. This also could be disastrous.

Dr. Semelweiss began the practice of washing his hands between patients. Yes, just that. The physicians of that time did not do this. In fact, most of the culture did not wash or bathe frequently. If you had to wash, you must be considered "dirty". The attitude of the physicians was that they were better than the ordinary man, and therefore they could not be considered dirty. It was an insult to be asked to wash, or to wash your hands. Arrogance deterred the necessary implementation of this vital practice.

Dr. Semelweiss persisted in washing his hands between patients. He instituted changing the water in the basin as well. He also began to use washed instruments before we knew about sterilization or wearing gloves. This important change saved the lives of many women and their babies. Dr. Semelweiss was ridiculed and ostracized for his belief. The medical doctors of his day were offended by his outrageous conduct, and he was shunned and jeered. His patients continued to find him after he was banned from his profession. Thankfully his reforms saved lives, transformed the practice of medicine and nursing, and transformed the healing arts for all time.

The mention of this historical reference has significance as an important medical reformation. Technology has enhanced medical progress. New surgical techniques are becoming available in rapid succession. The startling contradiction in all of this progress is our inability to control insulin resistance. It has taken two years to go from 61% to 65% in the obese insulin-resistant population. The reason for this increase is cited in the media as a lack of exercise, lack of willpower, and an inability to control portions. The medical and nutritional establishment will always offer the constant advice to exercise more, reduce calories, and to exert more will power. Often those who challenge this collective mind will be subject to severe criticism.

In recent collective memory, we can all remember the criticism aimed at Dr. Atkins. Many of his recommendations were his attempt to reform the way we relate to nutrition. It has taken years to vindicate some of his theories. Even now the work of Dr Atkins is being made politically correct by the need for balance and sensibility. It is being greened and fibered. For economic gain, the Atkins name has been associated with products that bear little connection to his theory. It is interesting to observe how individuals use the word "Atkins". It is commonly linked with a high-fat, low-carbohydrate eating style. Many other interesting styles of dieting behaviors and perceptions are included under the Atkins umbrella. Some of these styles of dieting rarely reflect what Dr Atkins intended.

# Why You Can't Have Your Cake & Eat It, Too

Often I am asked if I am putting forth an "Atkins-like" diet. The short answer is, "No." In all of the Atkins material I have read over the years I have not seen the subject of protein or water addressed. In all of the individuals I have worked with who have brought with them the knowledge of "Atkins", no two of them were doing the same thing. As universal as the name Atkins is, very different interpretations are applied. The interpretations reflect the perceptions. My work in developing a nutritional strategy is to open a channel for nutritional reform. As nutritional thinking is reformed, then true health reform can begin.

Standing in the way of these types of reforms is the food pyramid. In mythical terms it existed as a place of burial of kings. In a symbolic way it represented economic favoritism, and so does the food pyramid. It does not represent a way to provide human physiologic needs. It is not therapeutic or corrective for human nutritional problems. It does not maintain weight or health. The American Diabetic Association uses the concepts of the food pyramid in teaching diabetics about their nutritional needs. It is an amazing fact that diabetic patient's decline in health is directly linked to what she eats; yet the ADA continues with the concepts of high carbohydrates.

The Great Pyramids of Egypt rest on the banks of the Nile. So too do we try to deny or use denial to cover up these forms of favoritism or secret agendas. The call for nutritional reformation is long overdue. We cannot afford the weight. We cannot afford to wait.

# Why You Can't Have Your Cake & Eat It, Too

## Waiting to Exercise

The day will come when exercise will become a part of your wellness plan.  In part, this will be due to the loss of weight on the skeletal frame.  High blood pressure will be under control and fluid retention will be released.  You will feel strong and centered when you walk.  This can be a good time to begin a walking program.  One of the myths I hear about exercise is the problem of gaining weight due to increased muscle.  Remember, a pound is a pound.  A pound of muscle weighs the same as a pound of fat.  A pound of feathers weighs the same as a pound of steel.  The volume or the size of the mass is the only difference.

I remember a day when the summer Olympics were on TV.  A female weight-lifter weighed 103 pounds.  Her body fat was 7%. Surely she was strong.  I watched in amazement as she lifted 300 pounds.  The moral of this observation is; muscle doesn't have to weigh a lot to be powerful.  Develop the muscle you have, and you will improve the weight you carry.

First, we need to talk about aerobic exercise.  All of the so-called health segments on TV go on and on about the importance of regular exercise.  The point needs to be made for aerobic exercise, which is done with the inclusion of regular breathing.  This regular breathing means that oxygen is being exchanged in our lungs.  In order to insure we are getting enough oxygen to our heart and lungs during exercise we need to be working our heart at 75 to 50 percent of its maximum capacity.  How do we know what this means?

Maximum heart rate means the heart is operating at 100% of its anticipated capacity.  If the heart remains at its 100%

workload, it will become exhausted, and we do not want that to happen.  In aerobic activity, the heart is being worked gradually to 70% or less of its maximum rate.  To find out what your aerobic heart rate is, subtract your age from the number 220.  (The number 220 is the heart rate of a 21-year-old man who exercised to exhaustion.)  The result of that will represent your 100%, or your maximum heart rate in beats per minute.  Then multiply that sum by 75%, 65% and 55% to find your aerobic heart rates in beats per minute.  Keeping your heart rate in these percentages will mean that your body is able to get enough oxygen.  Getting adequate oxygen is important in insuring that the heart, lungs, and brain are being oxygenated during activity.  This aerobic quality is an insurance strategy you create in your body.  It means your body has enough oxygen to oxidize fat during the exercise of your choice.

Should one exceed the 75% heart rate in beats per minute, then the activity is anaerobic.  Anaerobic work is work without the presence of oxygen.  We wouldn't hold our breath and run a mile.  Yet, we see individuals who are breathless and working up a sweat, with little regard for the heart rate.  They may have the treadmill on its highest elevation while they are running.  Worse yet, they may be wearing clothing that causes them to overheat so they can lose fluid.  These are dangerous practices and are not helpful in oxidizing stored fat.

# Why You Can't Have Your Cake & Eat It, Too

Here is how you find out what your aerobic heart rate is:

220 - <u>Your age</u> = your 100% maximum heart rate (MHR)

100% MHR x <u>75%</u> = Your aerobic heart rate in beats
per minute

<u>100% MHR x 65%</u> = Your aerobic heart rate in beats
per minute

Here is a worksheet for you to make your calculations:

220 – (Subtract your age) = ___________
(Your 100% heart rate in beats per minute)

_______ - Your 100% heart rate X 75% = ___________
(Your 75% aerobic heart rate in beats per minute)

_______ - Your 100% heart rate X 65% = ___________
(Your 65% aerobic heart rate in beats per minute)

_______ - Your 100% heart rate X 55% = ___________
(Your 55% aerobic heart rate in beats per minute)

You can find your pulse or heart rate on your wrist, temple, or in the neck. Using your finger, palpate your pulse. Count for 30 seconds according to the second hand of your watch or stopwatch. Multiply that number by 2 to give you your pulse rate for 60 seconds. Do not use the thumb, as it has a pulse and will interfere with the count.

# Why You Can't Have Your Cake & Eat It, Too

Remember, your aerobic work will last only as long as you exercise. Once you stop, the effect ceases. Your purpose in doing regular exercise needs to change. Most of the time you have been using working out as a way to lose weight or to maintain your weight. It will do neither.

The most important reasons to do regular exercise are:

- To improve coordination

- To improve the immune system

- To improve the stress response

- To process stress

- To improve sleep

- To provide weight-bearing activity

- To get outside of the house!

There is a lot of mysticism about the word "metabolism." In the collective mind, metabolism is thought to be the energy that utilizes calories and even burns up fat. Many times, as a way to rationalize why we have gained weight, it will be suggested that our metabolism has decreased. This rationale suggests that this slowdown in metabolism is due to age, sickness, or the dreaded change of life. First, we analyze. Second, we paralyze. Then, the resistance begins. We've got to speed it up, got to go faster, and got to work harder.

The reality of the chemistry of food and its impact on your body is the single causative factor in fat oxidation.

# Why You Can't Have Your Cake & Eat It, Too

In order to increase muscle mass by ten pounds, one must lift weights. However the effort required doing this will require six months of lifting weights eight hours a day. The additional ten pounds of mass only requires 75 calories. This is a piece of bread!

While I would agree that maintaining a vital muscle mass is important for the creation of health, it can be done simply and inexpensively. The difficulty is in maintaining it. If one doesn't exercise for two weeks, then all the gains in muscle conditioning are lost. It is start-over time. This is the rule and not the exception. Life is full of starts and stops. It is just the way it is. Quitting is not an option. Fortunately, if the diet is consistent (high-protein low-carb moderate fat), then weight will not be regained. That is the hard part.

The reality of weight management is that it is work.

## Chapter 9:
## Changing the Way You Look at Change

### The Love Birds

One hot day last summer we experienced a very strong dust storm, preceding a very severe thunderstorm.  In the desert, we welcome the rain.  Summer heat is relentless here, and rain is something we long for.  This time, as usual, the power went out, the house was plunged into darkness and the air conditioning went off.   We waited it out, turning on our flashlights; lighting candles would be too hot.  We listened to a scanner to learn about the goings-on in the community.  Trees were blown down, blocking the roads.  One house sustained a direct lightning strike and was burned to the ground.  This was a big storm.

Soon  power was restored.  Fortunately we had shut down the air conditioner so the surge of power wouldn't overload the compressor.  After a few more minutes, we turned the air conditioner back on.  There was nothing more to do, but wait out the rain, which was coming down in wonderful torrents.

The next morning when I was at the kitchen sink, making coffee, I saw four lovebirds all huddled together on the window ledge looking mournful and battered.   They were grouped into two pairs, and had the typical markings of peach colored faces and green wings.  The underbellies were blue. They looked like little parrots. I immediately grew concerned for their safety.  Had these birds been released? Had they escaped captivity during the storm?  Surely, whoever owned them, I reasoned, would want to have them back.  Would these domesticated birds be able to survive in the "wild?"

## Why You Can't Have Your Cake & Eat It, Too

It was already 90 degrees at 8:00 a.m., and I had visions of these little creatures dying of dehydration in my yard. I worried about the local tabby cat that did surveillance on my back porch, imagining her with green feathers hanging from her jaws and the lovebird impaled on her claws. There were no lovebird food nibbles in my yard. I didn't have a feeder or a birdbath. What would I do? Surely, a rescue would fit the bill. I had to get birdseed right away.

With it getting hotter by the hour, I felt I had to act swiftly. Off to the local pet emporium, I made haste. Mind you, I didn't have a plan, but no matter. I was certain I would think of something. I began to peruse the aisles with a shopping cart. I found a bird feeder, a watering dish, and some wild birdseed (Twenty pounds – would that be enough?), some peanut butter birdseed cakes that required a special device to hold them, and a lovebird book so that I would be knowledgeable about them. I bought everything. Then I had a one of my grand ideas. I found a cage suitable for containing the lovebirds.

I hadn't caught them, but I was planning to do just that very thing. After all, how could they survive another minute without my intervention? I drove directly home with all this stuff and began the assembly of my rescue and capture. With the birdbath hung and the feeders stocked, birds of all feathers were enjoying the feast. The lovebirds had left the yard at some point. I was certain they had succumbed.

My son, who is an engineer, was recruited to help me make a lovebird snare. We stocked the birdcage with all kinds of lovebird treats and perches. We devised a complex system of pulleys using fishing line, to close the cage at the precise moment the lovebirds went inside. Then we hung the cage near the area where the lovebirds were last seen, and waited. We tested the pulley system on the cage and it worked well from inside the house. Technology is wonderful. We had a plan.

Just before dark, the lovebirds returned to my tree outside the kitchen window. I froze, poised with my hand on the fishing line. I guess I was fishing for lovebirds. The four lovebirds fed themselves, and drank the water. I was relieved. They were alive. Soon there were four more lovebirds in the tree, yammering for a spot on the bird feeder. Now we had four pairs. It was a beautiful sight.

I waited with the expectation that a lovebird would get into the cage. At that moment, I planned, I would close the door, and I would have rescued one bird. Then what would I do? Lovebirds are pairs. I couldn't separate them. If I had two lovebirds in the cage at one time, would it be the right pair? I needed to think about this.

I had birds as pets inside the house at one time. I remember how noisy they were and how much mess they made. One year on Easter Sunday a parakeet flew into an open window here. It was tame, and we kept it for a long time. We called it Easter.

I got out the lovebird book I had bought earlier, and decided I needed to learn a little more about the captive habits of lovebirds. Then I called a friend who I knew was knowledgeable about birds. By now I was realizing that I was signing myself up for a lot of work. No matter, I reasoned. I would capture the birds and turn them in to the pet store. Then they could be sold to homes, and be saved. I waited and waited. Days went by. Weeks went by. The lovebirds came and went. I kept the feeders full, and refilled the water. I looked forward to their visits.

Of course, by this time birds of all feathers were feeding in the yard. Finches of all colors, doves, quail, and the dreaded pigeons were helping themselves to the food. When the lovebirds made the scene, they were bossy and raucous. They squawked at the other birds to get the best spot in the feeder. This was getting interesting. The lovebirds were bullies. They were getting along just fine.

They did not need my help. This came as a shock to me. Why did I think I had to do something? My plan was a good one. It had been about six weeks, and not one of the lovebirds had entered the cage. I was not even close to getting one or a pair. Then I changed.

I noticed how much I enjoyed the birds feeding outside my window. The lovebirds came twice a day making a big scene out of pushing all the other birds away. It was delightful to see how the pecking order worked. I didn't have to capture the birds. They captured me. They were free and so was I. There was no need to separate the pairs and sell them into some form of pet slavery. I didn't have to clean cages and change paper. I had the joy of expecting their visit. I took their pictures. I have a video of all eight of them.

The summer continued, and the marauding tabby cat made the back yard unsafe. The lovebirds didn't come back. All of the other birds took their chances.

# Why You Can't Have Your Cake & Eat It, Too

I walk a mile and a half route around the neighborhood, each morning very early.  Months went by, and then I spotted the lovebirds.  They had taken up with someone else!!  At first I was envious, but soon I remembered how much joy they had given me.  I marveled at the wisdom of nature.  It was someone else's turn to tend them.  It wasn't about me.

The lovebirds taught me a couple of things.  One thing for sure, I needed to be patient.  I learned that the universe worked perfectly and it didn't need my help.  It was not about me.  Then I felt very lucky.  I had been given eight lovebirds and  I didn't have to pay for them.  All I needed to do was supply birdseed and water.  With patience, they would return.  I waited.

Sure enough, the first week in July they returned.  First there was just one.  The old worrier got activated.  Then there were two.  I was happy.  Then there were four, and today there are six.  After a month, we counted nine lovebirds.  Perhaps the delay in the arrival of a baby kept them away.

Fortunately for me, I became willing to change my point of view.  Once I realized the prize nature had given to me, it was up to me to accept it just the way it was.  It was odd to see them in the highest  palm tree after seeing them on perches in cages in a pet store.

The lovebirds were just like the rest of the wild birds, only prettier and more entertaining.  I have also been told that many lovebirds have found their way into local areas.  They congregate in packs in several locations. This taught me another thing - I  am not the only one who is lucky.

## Why You Can't Have Your Cake & Eat It, Too

Many people purchase pets of all kinds, but for one reason or another, the pet does not  always fit the lifestyle of the owner. With birds, fish, and cats being such self-sufficient creatures, they are often abandoned into the area.  So I had  reasoned that these lovebirds were released at some point.  The miracle is, they survived.  The second miracle is, they visit me a couple of times a day during the summer.  The third miracle is, I learned to accept the gift.

There I was one day, planning to take over the lovebird population in my yard and turn them in to a pet store.  Then I chose to change the way I saw this wonderful opportunity.  I changed my worldview.   One of the things the lovebirds taught me was that what I wanted was very different from what I needed.  My notion that  this generous gift of nature should be captured and put in a cage just didn't match reality. They could exist just the way they  were right now.

The second thing I learned from my experience was how my perceptions could expand and change.  The instant I viewed the birds as being capable of surviving on their own, both of us were free.  Had I continued to pursue my need to capture and control them, I could have created a lot of unnecessary suffering.  The birds would have been separated and I would have to provide them with a home.

The third thing I learned was that contentment and satisfaction could  be  experienced  as  an  observer  rather  than  as  a participant.  Perhaps my best role was to be the observer.

# Why You Can't Have Your Cake & Eat It, Too

I needed to relinquish my stubborn attitudes about helping the lovebirds. They had helped me immensely by just being there.

Learning something from such an unexpected source was a surprise. In order to enjoy my birds, I needed to change my attitude. It also occurred to me that I was changing my perception. Stubbornness is one of my favorite character flaws and has given me some of my best life lessons. Stubbornness is like resistance. Could there be a relationship between stubbornness and disease? Could rigidity in attitudes create rigidity in the body?

Today we are looking at the mind-body-spirit inter-connection. This inter-being, as it is now called, means our emotional resistance shows up in the body as a state of <u>dis-ease</u>. Intellectual refusal could be resistance. Apathy is resistance. This was and is all too interesting for me to contemplate.

Creating a stream of healthful living for the birds and me required a change in my belief system. My belief systems had convinced me that in order to do something right, I had to do it myself. Clearly, I was being shown by the lovebirds that they were doing something very right. They didn't need my interference at all. When I let go of my need to fix things, I found myself enjoying the natural order of my backyard bird show.

As a result of this experience, I felt compelled to write a poem, which I chose to title "Space." The space to which I am referring has to do with the fraction of time between perception and action. This relationship is usually measured in seconds, minutes, or hours. I chose to change the

# Why You Can't Have Your Cake & Eat It, Too

measurable dynamic from a time to an experience, the experience of grace.   Grace can be luck, a pause, or Divine Intervention.  However it shows up, is up to us.

One day I saw the lovebirds as being helpless and neglected. The next day I saw them as wonderful and capable.  I just added the seed.


## Space

Missions of Courage into the Night
Dark thunderheads loom
Winds drive the dust
Rain bringing its gift to the light.

Lightning crackles, slicing the air
Visions of the distant mountains
Rolling swirling clouds
This is Nature's dancing affair.

White-tailed doves sit in the trees
The ravens glean the shade
Lizards hanging from the eaves
Cicadas humming louder than bees.

A moment of pause, brief quiet space
Challenge to the senses
A signal, a pattern, holding
Waiting, watching the Breath of Grace.

## Chapter Ten:
## Insulin Resistance

### What does it mean?

Often I ask my patients with adult-onset diabetes to tell me what they think this diagnosis means.  Without exception they state that they have developed diabetes because their pancreas has stopped producing insulin.   In the many interviews with these patients, only one person said that the diabetes developed because she was allergic to sugar.  This answer is very close to the truth. When the tissues reject insulin they also refuse the sugar carried with it.  This process resembles an allergy.  In medical terminology we say this is an autoimmune response.  The popular perception that the pancreas has quit working is not true.  In most cases the pancreas is over-functioning because insulin is meeting specific tissue resistances.

For years we maintained a sugar embargo against Cuba where they kept producing sugar, loading it on boats, and attempting to cross into American waters, only to be sent back by our United States Coast Guard.  This is a specific type of resistance.  In addition, the United States had a blockade around Cuba to prevent needed food, medicine and materials from reaching this island.  This type of resistance restrained the Cuban people for years.   Meanwhile, Americans were able to obtain sugar and other goods from many places around the world.  Cuba was not.  Its commerce and culture regressed during these years of embargo.

# Why You Can't Have Your Cake & Eat It, Too

Perhaps this is a strange analogy, but it does illustrate resistance. Think of insulin resistance as a type of cellular embargo. The insulin resistance acts like the Coast Guard preventing goods from going in or going out. The body gets the role of Cuba. Consider how long it took for the infrastructure of that society to break down. Some of us are just as unlucky.

We now recognize that there are specific areas of the body that have become insulin-resistant, -- namely, muscles and fat. In some individuals the muscles are insulin-resistant and the fat is not. In others the fat is insulin-resistant and the muscles are not. And there are also some individuals who have insulin-resistance in both areas. Also, we must not underestimate genetics in the development of insulin-resistance. The addition of a genetic component is the wild card in the tendency to develop insulin resistance. As confusing as this might be, it is the best understanding we have at this moment in time.

Abdominal fat is located in the visceral compartment and is insulin-intolerant. That is the best way to think about it. Imagine fat packed in bundles around the vital organs located there. Consider the fat storage on the intestinal wall, under the diaphragm, wrapped around the liver, and packed around the spleen. This fat is known to repel insulin. This type of fat is insulin-repellent. The longer it resides in the body, the clearer its signal to all the cellular tissues, so that they in turn begin to repel insulin.

Sometimes normal-weighted people become insulin-resistant and go on to develop disease due to insulin resistance of the muscles. So one doesn't have to be fat to get this syndrome.

# Why You Can't Have Your Cake & Eat It, Too

Insulin resistance is an adaptation our bodies have made in response to the continuous exposure to carbohydrates of all kinds and the insulin needed to mediate them.

Think of this insulin-repellent activity like mosquito repellent. Even the best insect repellent will lose its strength after a few hours. Eventually insulin resistance is worn down by the bombardment of insulin and sugar. At this point in time the blood sugar may shift downward or go dangerously high. Usually by this time the intake of food has resumed, and the blood sugar insulin drama gets going one more time. It is a repeating cycle accompanied by feelings of fatigue and hunger. Sometimes there is muscle pain. At this time we must remember how hungry the body is for nourishment.

Another way I like to look at this is through analogy. In a scene from the move "Catch Me If You Can," Leonardo Di Caprio is looking through the window of his remarried mother's home on Christmas Eve. He sees the decorations and gifts under the tree. There is food on the table. A little girl is looking at him through the window. Suddenly she says to her mother that she sees someone out there. Di Caprio runs away. He knows something has changed and he recognizes he can't go there. He cannot be nourished in the same way. He cannot go home and be welcome.

This little excerpt symbolizes insulin resistance. The elements of nourishment are just beyond our grasp. They are there. We know it. Nourishment cannot come through the window. There is nothing we can do to get at it. We retreat in pain, walking around hungry for something.

## Why You Can't Have Your Cake & Eat It, Too

Sometimes this Insulin repellent can become very strong. The strong insulin-rejection response of the cells is in proportion to the amount of force exerted by the abdominal fat or the muscle. This may seem a confusing paradox, but it is worth attempting to understand. All carbohydrate will become sugar as it reacts in the human body. Once this digested sugar permeates the blood it becomes blood sugar. This is true in all of humanity, whether one has diabetes or not. Blood sugar requires a pancreatic insulin response. As rapidly as the pancreas produces insulin to bind to blood sugar, the insulin-repellent starts its reactance. This will be the case in those with predisposed insulin-resistant cellular behaviors. Remember, the pancreatic insulin prohibits the body from using its fat reserves as long as the sugar and insulin are in suspension. Insulin inhibits stored fat from being used and must be secreted in sufficient amounts for carbohydrates to be disposed. This creates delay. It is weight. It is wait.

As in the game of chess, it becomes an endless game of check and checkmate. Imagine playing the game of "Tic-Tac-Toe" and always playing to a cat game. This is another way to look at the phenomenon of insulin resistance and rejection. The pancreas is a very serious, hard-working devoted organ. It will not reduce its insulin production until there is reduction in blood sugar. The slightest encouragement given to the pancreas in its effort to reduce blood sugar will be noted in the Insulin embargo of the body. The insulin-resistance will be ready next time, but in double capacity.

As the fat mass expands, insulin production keeps up the same pace. The insulin rejection, the blood sugar and fat accumulation continue. Muscle insulin-resistance will also become more reactive. The blood sugar level, as noted on a blood test, will be dangerously elevated. In everyday speech someone might say, "Oh, my doctor told me I have sugar." If we really had the depth of understanding necessary, we would see that the blood insulin is also dangerously elevated. These two values are congruent for a time. The pancreas will secrete insulin until its supply is exhausted.

Think of this as being an oil well. One day there are 100 barrels a day, and suddenly nothing. Are we developing efficient energy systems? Are we trying to find alternative sources of fuel? While our society races against the clock to find sources of energy, can we see some signs that apply to the health of our country?

To illustrate this point, consider the rubber band. A rubber band is stretched and contracted many times in the course of its "life." At some point it begins to have a loss in its elasticity. There may be microscopic cracks in the rubber. Then one day it snaps, and it cannot be put back together. The cracks in our rubber band represent symbolically the markers of insulin resistance. Those "cracks" are obesity, high blood pressure, high LDL cholesterol, high triglycerides, gastro-esophageal reflux, fluid retention, irritable bowl syndrome, Fibromyalgia, and gout.

Remember, just one of those items can be a sign of impending adult onset diabetes.

In these circumstances, eliminating the need for pancreatic insulin will reduce insulin resistance. Until the body begins to heal from the consequences of hyper-insulinemia and glucose toxicity, restriction of glucose containing foods will be necessary.

The reduction of pancreatic insulin production will enable the body to release its fat stores.. As the fat storage is utilized for energy, the fat mass is reduced in size. Reduction of the insulin embargo will allow for the unrestricted nourishment of the body's hungry cells from your fat reserves. Energy is obtained from stored energy in the fat reserves. This energy provides a high caloric value, is easily renewed and can be quickly converted to power in the absence or restriction of insulin.

Stored fat contains tremendous caloric value. A pound of fat is worth 3,500 calories. If the patient has 100 pounds of excess fat, the caloric value is 350,000 calories. If he can utilize 2,000 calories per day, this 100 pounds of fat will last 175 days.

Body fat is important to maintain, but at a lesser amount. As we age, our body fat ranges differ. Also, men and women differ in the appropriate body fat percentages. Women who maintain a 35-40 pound fat mass can find it maintainable. Men can maintain a 20-30 pound fat mass without much difficulty. The important issue here is, what are the physical findings?

Try to remember that the insulin embargo will not go away. It is unresponsive to the political climate in the world. It will emerge again once carbohydrate eating is resumed. This is like the allergic response. Allergies are systemic, residing in the whole of the body. Pollens, poison ivy, and cat dander are examples of common allergens. The more one is exposed to these things, the more explosive the allergic response. If one is able to eliminate the exposure to the allergens, the auto-immune reaction capability is there but not needed. This is the way it is with insulin resistance.

By eliminating glucose-containing nutrients, insulin is not needed and the embargo factor is not required. Restricted glucose-nutrient exposure may still require pancreatic insulin. This means that eating little amounts of carbohydrate may cause an over-stimulation of insulin. One will have to evaluate the significance of the symptoms and the obesity to determine what the proper level of dietary carbohydrates should be, if any. Protein and water intake must be maintained.

It is true that the majority of late-onset diabetics are over-fat, with high blood pressure, elevated cholesterol, and gastro-reflux disease. These are the most frequently noted symptoms of emerging diabetes, although there are others. It is also true that a minority of late-onset diabetics are normal-weighted with one or more risk factor, plus a family history of late-onset diabetes. In both scenarios, the emerging diabetic is facing progression of this disease due to blood sugar elevations.

Prolonged blood sugar elevations result in tissue destruction. Elevated blood sugar means that nutrients are stalled in suspension in the blood. Elevated blood sugar means suspended nutrients are unable to be utilized by all the living tissues in the body. Those hungry muscles, organs, eyes, or kidneys will turn on themselves to get the essential nutrient: protein. When this scenario progresses in the diabetic, we see kidney destruction, blindness, and ulcers of the legs and feet.  Blood pressure elevations most certainly parallel blood sugar elevations.  The results of prolonged elevations in blood pressure are dangerous.  This perception is correct.

The perplexing problem in managing the diabetic patient is directly connected to effective blood sugar/insulin management.  This can be managed by carbohydrate correction to the diet, but it rarely happens that way.  Effective nutrition for the diabetic requires planning, accountability, shopping, and real-time preparation.  This means one will have to shop, plan meals, cook, and clean.

This work is so very important.  Sometimes we get so caught up in the results that we let judgment, comparison and fear sidetrack us.  We lose sight of the process.   These are bits of emotional resistance coinciding with our physical resistance, and there are always others.

Coincidentally, the weight reduction diet will require the same elements and effort.  It is interesting to note that both conditions respond in a positive way to an increase in protein, a decrease in carbohydrates, a moderate intake of fat, and liberal amounts of water.  It is an individual plan.  This is flying solo.  You must do it for yourself  and you must do it every day .

Remember, our physicians, nurses, and other allied professionals are helpful in diagnosing, educating, and following up on our care when we are sick.  The rugged individualism that founded this country doesn't exist in health care. The pioneering spirit that said, "I can do it" is giving way to "Let someone else do it for me".  A recent commercial says apathy is lethal. We are facing a serious, deadly foe with the capacity to maim and kill. This disease is insulin resistance.

**The accomplishment becomes the seedling of self-worth.**

Traditional nutritional education it is loaded with half-truths and fear-based marketing. Nutritional chemistry is the most significant element of diabetic and obesity recovery. Yet the way the chemistry is structured and taught insures progressive disease and weight increase. When traditional nutrition is encountered in the clinical management of the diabetic, its source is the standard American Diabetes Association training program. This plan prescribes the food pyramid, limiting portions, counting exchanges, counting calories, and exercise as the means to provide blood sugar management. As mentioned earlier in this work the typical content of the ADA diet will be 500 grams of carbohydrates, a deck-of-cards-size portion of protein (60 grams, and very little fat (20 Grams). Water intake is rarely addressed. This results in dehydration, protein depletion, out-of-control blood sugars, increase of symptoms, and increasing body size.

Even more disturbing is the trend of attending weekly weight loss group meetings for the weigh-ins and discussions. I have reviewed the menus they suggest in their monthly magazine. A typical day will provide 320 grams of carbohydrates, 60 grams of protein, and 30 grams of fat. For those with insulin resistance, this is just as deadly as the ADA formula. A large food manufacturer owns this particular weight-loss group. It is in their own best interest to recommend the serving sizes and foods. Why would they suggest that their group members restrict anything?

# Why You Can't Have Your Cake & Eat It, Too

The physician may prescribe insulin injections or oral medications to lower blood sugar.  Blood sugar management with the ADA regimen will lead to the gradual increase in blood sugar and increasing insulin resistance.  Diabetes education has its emphasis on avoidance of low blood sugars by the continuous feeding of carbohydrates.  There is just as much to fear from a low blood sugar as a high blood sugar.
The health provider will begin delivering the lecture series I like to think of as 'OR ELSE!"  It will go something like: "You had better get these blood sugars under control or else....".  Then there is this one: "You are gaining so much weight, I am going to have to do something drastic.... or else!"  In your defense you are doing just what you were told to do, most of the time.  You are using the carbohydrates to cover your medications or you are using the medicines so you can eat carbohydrates.

Off you go to the bookstore. A collection of cookbooks, books on diabetes and health will begin to fill the shelves at home, creating further confusion.  Again and again, these so-called health books propose portion control, the food pyramid, and exercise as the way to control diabetes.  Many times the individuals see themselves requiring more medical intervention for the newly developing symptoms. The blood sugar is out of control.  They may be noticing they are gaining weight at an alarming pace.  Worse yet, they may notice they are losing weight and don't know why.  Perhaps visual disturbances are noted as a result of high blood sugar levels in the vitreous fluids in the eye. There is protein excreted from the kidneys.  What has begun is the gradual disintegration of vital tissues.

# Why You Can't Have Your Cake & Eat It, Too

## Destruction appears because of prolonged blood sugar blood insulin and the insulin repellent response.

Diabetes represents a systemic refusal to accept the insulin produced by the pancreas. Remember, insulin has two purposes. One purpose is to move glucose into the tissues of the body, thereby lowering blood sugar. The other purpose is to signal the body to maintain or hold onto its fat stores. When there is a large secretion of blood insulin, everything stalls. Fat will be stored as fat, dietary protein will not be used, and carbohydrates will remain deadlocked with insulin.

When fat intake falls below 10 grams per day, the liver will convert blood sugar into fat, the only circumstance causing this reaction. The typical diet offered by the American Diabetic Association's food guidelines and the food pyramid is a diet abysmally low in protein and water, with large amounts of carbohydrates, and very low in fat. For as long as I have been in nursing, this formula has not changed. It is clearly an example of doing the same thing in the same way and expecting a different result. It makes no physiologic sense, yet we do it over and over.

Diabetes occurs when the pancreatic insulin is unable to reduce blood sugar. The pancreas does not quit producing insulin in late-onset diabetes, although pancreatic exhaustion does occur much later on in the disease process. Until pancreatic exhaustion occurs, the pancreas is producing large quantities of insulin. A normal-weighted non-diabetic person will need only a small amount of insulin to maintain blood sugar, whereas the diabetic will require 10 times the amount of pancreatic insulin to stubbornly budge the blood sugar down from its elevated state.

# Why You Can't Have Your Cake & Eat It, Too

## What to do?

For the diabetic, finding a compatible eating strategy is imperative.  This can be done with food available in the marketplace and with food that complements individual food preferences. Incorporating appropriate amounts of protein and fat must be started quickly, in order to provide the essential protein the body must have re-supplied each and every day. Fat intake must  be maintained to provide energy reserves and reassure the body that it will not starve.  Carbohydrates of all types must be limited, sharply.  Most importantly of all, water intake must be increased to three quarts per day, or at the very least, sustained at two quarts per day. Your liver will thank you for doing this.   Vitamins and minerals are also important to furnish micronutrients for the diet, as these are not obtainable in sufficient amounts from the food supply in existence today.

Do not fear eating protein.  Such fear is a cultural idea that has no basis in scientific fact.  This fear of eating protein, combined with the low-fat high-carbohydrate eating style is a formula for obesity and disease.  A long time ago, when there were range wars out on the prairie, farmers would be pitted against ranchers. These conflicts might put the sheep farmers against the pig farmers, and the cow farmers against the goat farmers.  The market today still reflects these prejudices.

Part of the misinformation we have been fed tells us that red meat contributes to overall cholesterol elevations. What must be considered in this assessment is what the exact food consumption is in an individual who is said to have high cholesterol.  He may eat red meat, but is it combined with

# Why You Can't Have Your Cake & Eat It, Too

French fries, chips, candy and sugar-loaded soft drinks? He may have had eggs, but were they included in a meal of pancakes, hash browns, and a big glass of orange juice? To affix blame on one food is like listening to one lung. We have to look at the whole milieu of nutrition. The contribution that the carbohydrate makes to the overall health picture is and has been discounted and minimized.

There are important market forces that depend on manipulating the food supply. Everyone wants his or her product to have preferential treatment in the marketplace. The manufacturers present their biases masqueraded as fact. One might conclude that the beneficiaries of this food misinformation would be the drug companies. Consider the number of obesity-related prescription remedies. Of course the food industry benefits. It is important that commerce is successful for the economy; yet, look at the cost to the consumer (increased illness) and to industry (increased health care costs passed on to the consumer).

## Children of the World

We have only to look around us. Children are developing late-onset diabetes and high blood pressure. Youngsters are entering puberty earlier and earlier. It is not unusual to hear about a 9-year-old weighing 100 or more pounds. The Wall Street Journal recently published an article on pediatric Bariatric surgery. Yes, teenagers are getting their stomachs stapled. The diet histories of youngsters are astonishingly abundant in carbohydrates. This high-carbohydrate cultural alignment is also a non-cooking culture. We must "have it now," in the greatest amount possible, and with the least amount of preparation. Alarmingly, youngsters are consuming cereal, milk, yogurt, bagels, pizza, fries, and chips in unlimited portions. Protein is omitted because it would have to be cooked. They have been raised on soda pop and they get little pure water. These youngsters are getting fat first and sick second. They become targets of abuse by their peers.

## Off the Soap Box and into the Elbow Grease

Blood sugar can be controlled with a high-protein low-carbohydrate diet and necessary medical intervention. This is possible by limiting your intake of carbohydrates to 50 grams or less every day. Protein intake must be increased to 1.5 grams of protein per kilogram of ideal body weight, which is a minimum level, but still far below what most individuals consume, if they eat any at all. To calculate your minimum levels of essential protein, refer to the section on "The Importance of Protein". Another way to calculate protein need is to allow one ounce of protein for each ten pounds of ideal body weight.

The body needs protein, and it can be consumed in large amounts without harm to the systems of the body. Holding to the levels suggested above will mean consuming at least 90 grams of protein every day. It just so happens that a high-protein low-carbohydrate diet will provide fat, but will be low in calories. This will decrease the body's need for pancreatic insulin and enhance the body's ability to utilize its fat reserves. This is how we were engineered.

With this simple plan, blood sugars will come down. As they do, it will be important to develop a sliding scale to adjust your medications. It doesn't make sense to take insulin and oral hypoglycemic agents when the blood sugar is stabilizing downward.  Stay in touch with your doctor for guidance in this matter.  It also doesn't make sense to use juice or candy to elevate blood sugar when medications are being used for control of blood sugar.  Using candy or frosting on the gums will raise your blood sugar, but you will feel the effects of these huge swings in energy.  It will set off the hyper insulinemic response and the resulting insulin immunity.  It is better to decrease your need for medications by decreasing your intake of all carbohydrates.

Most important, do not take your insulin and skip meals.  Of course the blood sugar will stay down or even bottom out, but this is a very dangerous practice. Some people use this type of planning to allow for intentional continued use of candy. Candy maintenance is a practice used by some diabetics to manage their blood sugar.  This keeps the blood sugar maintained, but the danger to the body cannot be averted.

Restricting your carbohydrate intake, increasing the protein intake, drinking lots of water, and maintaining a daily record will help you connect the dots between blood sugar and carbohydrate intake.  This continual link will give you the information you need to reduce your weight, reduce your blood sugar with the diet, and reduce the medications you are taking.  A medical professional must supervise this change. He will provide you with a sliding scale for your medications.

# Why You Can't Have Your Cake & Eat It, Too

**Some strategies to manage a low blood sugar:**

- Use a cracker with slices of ham and cheese or peanut butter.

- A couple of hard boiled eggs

- Celery with cheese sticks and cherry tomatoes

- Incorporate a dense low-carb fiber-like cracker with a dense protein, such as Ak-Mak, Kavali, or Wasa crackers with beef slices.

- A protein drink could be used.

- Meat jerky.

- Cottage or Ricotta cheese mixed with some peanut butter or sugar free Jell-o.

- A protein bar could be added as well; however, these bars will have a lot of carbohydrates.  Be attentive to those values.

- Keep these things ready while you go through this important work.

- Drink lots of water.

- Do not use juice, candy, fruit, or pastries.

This technique will be new to you.  In the past you have been instructed to have 30 grams of carbohydrates at each meal with a 30-gram snack in between.  This has kept the blood sugar high, requiring more medication.  The other instruction given is to add a large volume of carbohydrate when the blood sugar gets low.    Often this low blood sugar is hardly diagnostically low, and may be well within normal limits. But the individual may complain of feeling jittery, with the suggested fear that it will plunge lower. Pre-emptively, a high carbohydrate food will be ingested to take care of something that hasn't happened.    As a result the blood sugar goes higher.

There is damage done to the body when the blood sugar is too high, just as there is damage done when the blood sugar is too low.    With low blood sugars there is a loss of consciousness and function.  The destruction of a high blood sugar is hidden to us because our functioning or states of consciousness are not disrupted.   Make no mistake: high blood sugar is just as catastrophic as low blood sugar.

Feeling weak, jittery, or thirsty may be a good indicator for you.  Very often fatigue, nervousness, and thirst are ignored until it is too late.  Diabetics who skip meals, postpone needed rest, and don't want to be in the bathroom every hour resist the most necessary elements to health.  These elements are regular high protein meals, elegant periods of rest, and lots of water.

By utilizing the high-protein snack for the impending 'low sugar' episode, you will be providing your body the materials it needs to create sugar from the liver.  This maneuver will engage the liver in its own process of sugar production from the energy stores already in existence in your body.  It does work.  After a few times of practice with this technique it will be necessary to phone your doctor for instructions on medicine changes.  Soon you will have a blood test to check your blood sugar and the A1c.  At this time your patience and practice will be rewarded.

It doesn't make sense to continue eating large amounts of carbohydrates when one is a diabetic.  The body is rejecting this type of food.  This is what it means to be a diabetic.  A diabetic is allergic to carbohydrates.  For this patient, all carbohydrates must be limited continuously.

Stay in touch with your medical practitioner.  Keep accurate blood sugar and food records.  These records will act like a laboratory for you to observe your results parallel to the actions taken with food and medicine.  This will show you how your body is responding to the foods you eat and the medications you use for blood sugar control.  This is mathematics, science and effort combined.  It is not magic.

## Balancing the Paradigm

By now you may have begun to challenge the old dietary belief systems.  You may experience challenges to your program from various sources.

Could it be that the secret to improving your medical status and losing weight was giving up your intellectual and emotional resistance?

Could it be that your resistance to taking care of yourself is/was at the center of your diabetes?

Could it be that your energetic investment in your illness is greater than your investment in your health?

# Why You Can't Have Your Cake & Eat It, Too

Could it be that you are afraid of change?

Could it be you are as afraid to start, as you are afraid to stop?

How many times can the "dog eat your homework?"

These are questions that address the nature of behavioral resistance.  Stubbornness is resistance.  Think of it as intellectual or emotional resistance.  If we refuse to take our medicine or follow directions, then we delay our recovery.  We skip meals, take insulin, and eat candy.  We wait.  We weight.  Procrastination and justification are part of the same equation: resistance.

You are working on a miracle.  Miracles happen when science, math, and hard work are combined toward a specific goal.  Miracles do not resist, make excuses, cling to fears, create apathy, or procrastinate.

Balanced eating, portion control, counting calories, doing exercise has meant something very different from the ideas presented here.  Balanced, controlled caloric intake must reflect the physiology of nutrition as it appears in each individual.  The foods we utilize to recover our health and our body weight will have a balance and a rhythm to them, but will differ from our commonly held nutritional myths.  As mentioned often, we cannot have our cake and eat it too.  There is nothing better than  hard work, and you have to look before you leap.

## Appendix 1

### Preferred Reading List

<u>The Schwarzbein Principle Cookbook</u>, by Schwarzbein, DeVille, and    Jacob

<u>Everyday Low Carb Cooking</u>, Alex Haas

<u>500 LoCarb Recipes</u>, Dana Carpender

<u>15-Minute LoCarb Recipes</u>, Dana Carpender

<u>Atkins Best Recipes</u>, Time Life Publishers

<u>Finding Serenity in the Age of Anxiety</u>, Robert Gerzon

<u>The Nutribase Nutrition Facts</u>, Desk Reference

<u>Prayers for Healing,</u> edited by Maggie Oman

<u>The Dancing Wu Li Masters,</u> by Gary Zukov

<u>Power Versus Force,</u>  by David R. Hawkins, M.D.

<u>Blood Sugar Solution,</u> by Richard Bernstein, M.D.

## Appendix 2

## The Heart and Soul of the Program

Most diet books have a section where you can find the "guts" of the program, but many of the people who read these books start and stop with the program part of the book. They neglect to read the theory, including adjustments and difficulties that presented themselves during the development of the diet. Encounters with people who have "done" Atkins, South Beach, and the like have been very interesting. No two people "do" Atkins the same way, and this is true for the other programs. My impression is that the general concept of a program is usually the only idea that is taken away from the book. After that, the unfolding nutrition plan is imprinted with much nutritional mythology. The collective cultural nutritional mind always has the final say, it seems.

For a time, I thought I would camouflage the heart of the program in this writing. Sprinkling it here and there, it would force the reader to read the whole thing. Perhaps that would give the fullest exposure to these concepts, ensuring that the reader would know what to do and what to expect. So it is with reluctance that the heart and soul of my program is put in just one place. The menus and recipes are located nearby.

In the following twenty pages or so, you will find some limited food composition lists. Then you will have some work pages to figure out your personal dietary plan. This is not a one-size-fits-all program. Your particular eating plan must have items you will eat and must reflect your specific health concerns. Important issues such as travel, restaurant eating, and work must be considered as well.

# Why You Can't Have Your Cake & Eat It, Too

We are about to shift the energy.

**Protein Values**: 4 calories per gram

|  | Amount | Protein |
|---|---|---|
| Cheese | 1 oz | 9 gm |
| Lo-fat Cheese | 1 oz | 9 gm |
| Cottage Cheese | 1/3 cup | 10 gm |
| Egg | 1 | 6 gm |
| Egg whites | 3 | 10 gm |
| Egg substitute | 1/2 cup | 10 gm |
| Tuna h2o pack | 1 oz | 8 gm |
| Light white fish | 1 oz | 7 gm |
| Lobster/crab/shrimp | 1 oz | 6 gm |
| Salmon | 1 oz | 6 gm |
| Turkey breast | 1 oz | 8 gm |
| Chicken Breast | 1 oz | 8 gm |
| Beef lean | 1 oz | 9 gm |
| Pork Lean | 1 oz | 8 gm |
| Veal Lean | 1 oz | 8 gm |
| Lamb loin | 1 oz | 8 gm |
| Fat free deli meats | 1 oz | 5 gm |
| Jerky (varies by type) | 2 oz | 14 gm |
| Cream cheese | 1/4.cup | 10 gm |
| Ricotta cheese | 1/4.cup | 7 gm |

Please consult your food values book and read labels. These are cooked weights. The above is just a general guide. Remember that generally one-third of protein will contain fat. When in doubt, hunger, boredom or fear, eat protein.
Note: Protein caloric value is 1 gm protein = 4 calories

# Why You Can't Have Your Cake & Eat It, Too

| **Protein Substitutes** | Amount | Protein |
| --- | --- | --- |
| Mori NuTofu | 12.5 oz | 20 Gm |
| Morningstar Farms SW | 1 burger | 18 Gm |
| Morningstar Farms<br>   Quarter Prime | 1 burger | 24 Gm |
| Jerky Vegan | 1 oz | 14 Gm |
| | | |
| Pure Protein | 1 can | 20 Gm |
| Pure Protein | 1 can | 35 Gm |
| EAS Carb Sense | 1 can | 15 Gm |
| Atkins Protein Drink | 1 can | 15 Gm |
| Monster Protein Drink | 1 can | 50 Gm |
| | | |
| X Rated Protein | 1 scoop | 22 Gm |
| Whey Fuel | 1 scoop | 18 Gm |
| Designer Protein | 1 scoop | 18 Gm |
| Soy Protein | 1 scoop | 19 Gm |
| Ultra Plan | 1 scoop | 20 Gm |

These items represent high-protein low-carb protein drinks, substitutes, and powders.  Do not add fruit to them unless you have made room for them in your plan.  In most cases the protein powders should be blended with water or diet soda. There is a soymilk product called "Soy Slender" that is sugar free (not calorie free) that works nicely with the protein powders.

## Carbohydrates: 4 Calories Per Gram

**Fruit Category**          Carbohydrates in Grams

| Fruit Category | Carbohydrates in Grams |
|---|---|
| Apple   2 inch diameter | 14 |
| Applesauce 1/3 cup | 11 |
| Apricots   2 inch | 9 |
| Banana   ½ med. | 14 |
| Blackberries/blueberries ½ cup | 10 |
| Cantaloupe 1 quarter | 10 |
| Cherries 10 | 11 |
| Cranberries 1 cup fresh | 10 |
| Grapefruit half | 11 |
| Grapes 10 | 8 |
| Guava 2/3 | 10 |
| Kiwi | 11 |
| Nectarine | 9 |
| Orange small | 12 |
| Peach | 10 |
| Pineapple 1/8 fresh | 12 |
| Plums 2 | 12 |
| Strawberries 1 cup | 10 |
| Tangerine 1 | 12 |
| Watermelon 1 cup | 13 |

Problem fruits and fruit products include juices, and dried fruits.  They are notably very high in sugar content.  The list is just an overview on fruits.  Consult your food lists or call with questions.

# Why You Can't Have Your Cake & Eat It, Too

| Starch Category | Carbohydrates in Grams |
|---|---|
| Bread        1 oz | 20 |
| Bagel   1 oz piece | 20 |
| English muffin   half | 15 |
| Matzo      6-inch piece | 17 |
| Melba toast   5   pieces | 16 |
| Roll          1 oz | 20 |
| Tortilla    6-inch diameter. | 17 |
| Pita         half | 16 |
| Kavali crackers   4 | 16 |
| Wasa crackers   4 | varies by type |
| Rye crisp          4 | 16 |
| Lavosh      6 inch round | 10 |
| Macaroni, noodles, Spaghetti, 1/2  cup cooked | 20 |
| Rice          1/2  cup cooked | 30 |
| Beans, legumes 1/3   cup | 14 |
| Corn          1/2  cup | 16 |
| Parsnip          1/2 cup | 15 |
| Potato   1  medium | 17 |
| Sweet potato  1/4 cup | 21 |
| Pumpkin          1/2  cup | 10 |
| Yellow squash 3/4cup | 17 |
| Carrots          1 med raw | 7 |
| Tomato          2 small | 10 |

## Dairy Category

| | |
|---|---|
| Buttermilk      1 cup | 12 |
| Skim milk      1 cup | 12 |
| Yogurt nonfat 1 cup | 12 |

# Why You Can't Have Your Cake & Eat It, Too

| Vegetable category | | Carbohydrate in Grams |
|---|---|---|
| Asparagus | 1 cup | 4 |
| Broccoli | 1 cup | 4 |
| Bean sprouts | 1 cup | 5 |
| Green beans | 1 cup | 5 |
| Brussels | 1 cup | 10 |
| Cabbage | 1 cup | 6 |
| Cauliflower | 1 cup | 5 |
| Celery | 1 cup | 4 |
| Bok choy | 1 cup | 4 |
| Cucumber | 1 med | 4 |
| Eggplant | 1 cup | 8 |
| Endive | 20 leaves | 4 |
| Kohlrabi | 1 cup | 4 |
| Leeks | 1 cup | 3 |
| Lettuce | 3 ½ cup | 3 |
| Mushrooms 1/2cup cooked | | 4 |
| Onions | 1 cup raw | 12 |
| Green onions 1cup raw | | 6 |
| Peppers green, red  1/2cup | | 3 |
| Radishes | 12 | 4 |
| Sauerkraut | 1 cup | 5 |
| Spinach cooked 1cup | | 6 |
| Summer squashes 1/2 cup | | 3 |
| Turnips | 1 cup | 6 |
| Watercress | 1cup | 4 |

## Miscellaneous

| | |
|---|---|
| Oatmeal, plain 2/3 cup | 19 |
| White flour, 1    cup | 87 |
| Wheat flour,    1   cup | 87 |
| SUGAR, white 1   cup | 200 |
| SUGAR, brown 1-cup | 214 |

## Fat Category: 9 Calories to the Gram

| | | Fat per Gram |
|---|---|---|
| Canola Oil | 1 Tablespoon | 14 |
| Corn Oil | 1 Tablespoon | 14 |
| Peanut Oil | 1 Tablespoon | 14 |
| Olive Oil | 1 Tablespoon | 14 |
| Butter | 1 Tablespoon | 11 |
| Butter light | 1 Tablespoon | 6 |
| Cream H&H | 1 ounce | 4 |
| Cream Heavy | 1 ounce | 11 |
| Cream Light | 1 ounce | 6 |
| Margarine | 1 Tablespoon | 11 |
| Margarine Light | 1 Tablespoon | 6 |

## References

There are two major reference books, which can help you with your counts:

Nutribase Nutrition Facts is the most extensive reference book and it was used in the creation of these food lists.  It is available in most bookstores for under $26.  The program for computer databases made by the same company is available, and is priced at $650.  They have limited food compositions available for free online.

The Complete Book of Food Counts by Netter may also be helpful  It too is available in most bookstores for under $6.

Many of the references for food compositions are reflecting food counts in restaurants.  These change with the introduction of new products.  Be careful when reading food labels, so you can be sure the totals add up as given.

**Notes**

## Appendix 3

### The Right Fit

In order to get your nutritional formula, we have to address your body composition as you are right now.   Your age, height, and activity levels will be included in coming to a decision regarding your most appropriate ideal body weight. It will be hard to do, but try to let go of an old body image reminiscent of high school or college days. If you have approached this diet just like the others, you have said, "This time I'm going to get it right." "Right" just might be different.

Using the bio-impedance measurer we determined the body fat amount in pounds and percent.   By subtracting the estimated pounds of body fat from your current total body weight, we will have the amount of the lean body mass.  The lean body mass is zero percent body fat.  Try to remember it is important to have fat on the body.  If you had no fat, you would be starving, and using your own mass for food.  This is not healthful.

Men and women have differing needs as far as body fat mass is concerned.  Men can have variances in fat mass from 7% to 20%.  This means the fat mass weight could be 15 to 25 pounds of the total body weight.   Women can have variances in fat mass from 23% to 28%.  This means the fat mass could weigh 30 to 40 pounds.   These are examples of ways to address getting to your ideal body size.  First we have to know what your lean mass weighs.  If your lean body mass weighs 130 pounds, then your probable ideal body weight should be 165 pounds.   This is of course your decision.  We will want

# Why You Can't Have Your Cake & Eat It, Too

your ideal body weight to reflect your lean body mass plus an age/sex appropriate fat mass.  The purpose of this is to make certain we have an attainable and maintainable goal.

## Maintainable Goal Weight

Today's Date________________________

Your weights as you are today________________________

Bio-impedance:  Fat%____________ Fat pounds: __________

Current weight____________________

Minus fat #      ____________________

Lean body mass____________________

Add in age, sex, height appropriate, and activity appropriate fat mass in pounds____________________

Ideal body weight________________

## Now we can calculate your nutritional strategy.

## Protein Intake

Convert your ideal body weight into kilograms by dividing it by 2.2. (2.2 pounds per kilogram)

Ideal body weight _________divided by 2.2 = ____________kg.

# Why You Can't Have Your Cake & Eat It, Too

Next multiply your ideal weight in kilograms by 1.5 grams of protein to obtain your minimal protein need per day.

Kg ideal body weight _________X 1.5 gm Protein = __________

Another simple way to understand how much protein you need is to divide your current weight or your ideal body weight by ten.  For every ten pounds of ideal weight or maintenance weight, you will need one ounce of protein.

The key point is this: You can always increase your protein to maximum levels.  The minimum protein requirement is now established.

## Carbohydrate Intake

To plan carbohydrate elimination, start with a 2 to 1 ratio. Where the minimum protein intake is "2" and the maximum carbohydrate intake is "1." If your protein requirement is set at 120 grams, then the maximum carbohydrate intake will be half of that amount, or 60 grams.

If you have significant symptoms of insulin resistance, then you will have to reduce your carbohydrate intake to 50 grams or less.  This should disable your insulin resistance.  In most cases, this level will be effective in obtaining the results we want.  If it is not, then we must reduce the carbohydrate intake further.

Always keep the protein intake at the minimum levels or higher.  When in doubt, always eat more protein.

# Why You Can't Have Your Cake & Eat It, Too

Minimum Protein Intake ________________________ per day

Divided by 2 = Maximum carbohydrate intake ________ per day

## Fat Intake

Fat intake on the high protein diet has had a dubious history. The image of eating pounds of bacon swimming in fat, or drinking cream by the cupful, and drowning food in melted cheese is not what we are trying to achieve. Fat intake will be maintained, but at much lower levels.

Remember, we are not counting the fat in the meat, fish, pork, or poultry in the diet. We are looking at the fat in oil, butter, and salad dressings. Your fat intake while on the plan will be 75% of your maximum carbohydrate.

Carbohydrate intake ________ x 75% = ________ fat intake. These values are in gram weights. From the food lists we can convert the gram weight of something into pounds, ounces, or cups.

## Alcohol Intake

The key point about alcohol in the diet is to remember the body treats it like a fat. Weight loss seems to be retarded by alcohol intake. Avoid white wine, frozen concoctions, and beer. That leaves red wine, and the as we say the "hard stuff'. "

# Why You Can't Have Your Cake & Eat It, Too

Limit yourself to three glasses of red wine or 3 ounces of hard liquor a week.

If you do not use alcohol, there is no need to begin now!

## Water Intake

Water intake for everybody is 3 liters a day (96 ounces).  If you are very tall or have a lot of surface area, then increase your water intake to 4 liters a day.  If you are outside, be sure to drink lots of water.

## Vitamins and Minerals

Any good vitamin is fine.  It is not possible to get micronutrients from the food in our diet without consuming bushels of foods..  Vitamins are a good, non-caloric way to get essential nutrients.  Take one a day or use as directed.

Calcium supplements should be used as well.  Avoid those made from oysters or coral.  Use calcium supplements made from citrates, i.e. calcium citrate.  There are some suggested types in the shopping lists.

## Your Nutritional Prescription

Protein Intake per Day

Carbohydrates Intake per Day

Fat Intake per Day

Vitamins

Minerals

Water

**Daily Dietary Diagram  (Fill in amounts)**

Meal One

Protein

Carbohydrates

Fat

Meal Two

Protein

Carbohydrates

Fat

Meal Three

Protein

Carbohydrates

Fat

# Why You Can't Have Your Cake & Eat It, Too

## Blood Sugar Management 911 Kit

The purpose of this strategy is to elevate your blood sugar by using protein.  Please do not skip meals, and take your insulin or hypoglycemic medicines. This creates a terrifying blood sugar drop that is unnecessary. Skipping meals and taking your insulin or blood sugar-lowering prescriptions has a boomerang effect on blood sugar.  It may go low, but it will suddenly rise due to the stress response of the adrenal glands working with the liver.   Please avoid candy, sugar, or juice. Be certain your blood sugar is low by checking it.  Recheck the blood sugar after using these methods.

USE:

Protein Drinks
Jerky
Low Carb Bread with meat and cheese
Low Carb Cracker with meat and cheese
Low Carb Bread/cracker with cottage cheese
Low Carb Bread/cracker with cream cheese
Small fresh fruit with cheese or cottage cheese

Contact your medical provider for advice on changes to your insulin and/or oral hypoglycemic medicines.

## Stuffing the Shopping Cart

Vitamins - Daily multiple vitamin
Calcium - Caltrate D 1,000 mg per day
Fiber type bowel care-Fibercon tabs, Citrucel/Metamucil sugar free
Potassium Replacement-Emergence Lite

Protein suggestions:

Boars Head Deli Meats: Oven Roasted Turkey
Eye of Round Roast
Black Forest Ham
SnackMaster Jerky
Pacific Gold Jerky (Cost-Co)

Tuna in a bag: Look for foil bags in the canned meat section of your grocery.  There are many processed protein selections now prepared in foil packs. Look for turkey, chicken, and ham.

Protein Drinks: Pure Protein
Ultra Pure Protein Drinks
EAS Protein Drinks

Protein Powders: Whey Fuel
"X" rated
Soy Protein

Special Treats: Da Vinci Sugar Free Syrups
Mor-I-Nu Tofu

# Why You Can't Have Your Cake & Eat It, Too

Emergence-electrolyte drink: Potassium replacement

Here are some more items we might add to the list:

- Boar's Head Meats are found at Fry's Super Markets, Sunflower,  and some Basha's stores. Look for these items in your local grocer.

- Pure Protein, Robbins Nest Products are found at Hi-Health.

- Pure Protein is at Trader Joe's.

- Advantage protein drinks are widely available.

- EAS Carb Sense are also widely available at most grocery stores.

- Da Vinci Sugar Free Syrups and Walden Farms dressings are at specialty and health food stores

- SnackMaster Jerky is found at Whole Foods and Trader Joe's.

- Anything else?

## Appendix 4

## Special Conditions

It is with some reluctance that the following menu selections are included. I have often prepared specific menus for specific circumstances for specific individuals, and it occurs to me that creating menus can be helpful as a template or a frame for someone to use. On the dark side, menus can be used as another form of resistance. It is like creating the need for special conditions to be met in order for the task to be completed. As with anything, there are often special requirements.

This means the need to create special food, just the right thing, and the demands just keep on rolling. This is resistance. Yet, when I have done all of that for someone, I will hear him or her say, "Well, I just didn't have time to look at them." Or worse, "I just didn't like anything." Resistance. Of course, I waste no time in pointing this out to them. The whole idea is to show by example what can be done. It is experimentation with food types to put forward an exciting high protein, low carbohydrate, moderate fat eating plan. We are creating a plan with high nutrient value, a low pancreatic insulin requirement, and lots of fat lost.

I hope you enjoy some of the plans you have found here. Be sure to share your food plans with me. We can learn as much from the ones that worked as from the ones that didn't work.

# Why You Can't Have Your Cake & Eat It, Too

## Menu Strategies

<u>Morning</u>
2-4 Salmon Patties
Low-fat reduced-calorie Cilantro Dressing
2 Ak-Mak Crackers
2 Strips Bacon
1 quart water

<u>Snack</u>
Left over Salmon Patty

<u>Luncheon</u>
Grilled Tuna Salad Bowl
Romaine lettuces/green onion/ Marinated mushrooms (Trader Joe's)
½ cup chilled raspberries w/1 Tbsp cream
1-quart water/ Iced tea

<u>Snack</u>
2 Deviled eggs (use mustard, horseradish, capers)

<u>Evening</u>
Rack of Lamb
Marinated Asparagus (Trader Joes)
Iceberg Lettuce with small amount Bleu cheese dressing

Herbal tea

# Why You Can't Have Your Cake & Eat It, Too

<u>Morning</u>
4-6 ounces Tuna, drained
½  Red Pepper, sliced
1/8 fresh pineapple, slice
 2 Tbsp Ranch dressing
Water/Coffee

<u>Snack</u>
Celery Sticks & low fat cheese sticks

<u>Luncheon</u>
1-2 Roasted chicken breast, skinless (Boston Market)
Mixed Vegetables
Iced Tea/ Water

<u>Dinner</u>
4-6 ounces Eye of Round Roast Beef
Yellow crooked neck squash, grilled
Eggplant, grilled (spray with Pam, sprinkled garlic, balsamic vinegar)
Cucumber, Onion,  Peppers, 2 cherry Tomatoes
Oil & Vinegar garnish

Sweet Dreams

**Morning**

Turkey "Waldorf" salad:
       4 oz. Turkey Breast, bite size pieces
       1 cup fresh celery, chopped
       ½ apple, chopped
       Toss with rice vinegar and 1 tsp mayonnaise
2 Melba toast rounds, crumbled
16 oz Water /coffee

Luncheon
6-8 ounces Shrimp, chilled
Romaine lettuce, chopped green onion.2 cherry tomatoes
1 tbsp Ranch dressing, if desired
1 slice Kavali Crisp bread  (optional)
Iced Tea/water

Dinner
8 ounces Salmon, grilled
      Lemon Juice, capers,
4 hearts of artichokes (4)
1 cup fresh asparagus, steamed
1 tbsp butter
Mineral water

Recommended Daily Snacks Anytime:
Myo-Plex low carb protein drinks
SnackMaster turkey jerky or beef jerky
1-ounce cheese
Hard-boiled eggs
Boars Head Meat and Cheese

# Why You Can't Have Your Cake & Eat It, Too

<u>Morning</u>
3-egg Omelet w/chicken, cheese, peppers, onion, mushrooms
1 tbsp Salsa
Sour Cream
Guacamole
1 slice diet bread

<u>Lunch</u>
5 oz Chicken Breast, stir-fried w/ mushrooms, green beans,
Bok choi, ginger and garlic
Ginger and garlic
1 Tbsp oil

<u>Dinner</u>
8 oz Halibut
Red Peppers, grilled
5 Brussels sprouts, steamed and buttered
1 slice diet bread
Fresh plum w/ mint, chilled and sliced

96 ounces of water per day, vitamins

## Appendix 5

**Net Carbs**

Protein bars are also available for use in weight management techniques.   This item needs careful scrutiny.   In the manufacture of these products, many items, such as maltitol, glycerol and fiber are added to enhance the sweetness and the texture. Often these items are called non-impact carbohydrates and are excluded from the content label, as a marketing ploy. Remember, carbohydrates in any form impact blood sugar in all people.

Food labels aren't always truthful.  The total caloric count of an item may be correct, but the label can still show a disparity in the accounting of protein, carbohydrates, and fat.  Often these items are listed in gram weight without the caloric value listed.  This omission leads the consumer to believe that the item is a low carbohydrate food, which may not be the case. Remember, carbohydrates have four calories to the gram, as do proteins. Fat has nine calories to the gram.  In the very fine print it states the caloric value of sugar alcohol is 4.1 calories to the gram.

By multiplying the number of grams by the appropriate stated value, the amount of calories contributed by that item can be ascertained.   Adding those values, and subtracting that sum from the total stated caloric value can see the true values.  If there is a leftover caloric value it will show up in this accounting. Most often this leftover value is a carbohydrate.

To further illustrate this point, look at the new category "net carbs."  This value reflects the tally of the total carbohydrate count minus the fiber and sugar alcohol.  With consumers looking only at this "net carb" value they may feel at ease buying a product that contains a "net carb" value of 4 grams. The reality is that the low carb product may really contain a much higher food value than the stated label.  This has become a wide-open area in truth in labeling.  The food industry is trying to save itself in the marketplace.  The FDA has not looked at this new "net carb" designation.  In fact the FDA as admitted it has not had the time to fully absorb the "net carb" controversy into their proceedings.  Until they do, they have admitted it is every one for themselves.

For the low carb dieter, this is an area where even more self-discipline will need to be applied.   While we may crave chocolate ice cream in all of its sugar and fat, the low carb chocolate ice cream may seem very appealing.  Once the label is examined, it will yield the same approximate food value as the regular ice cream per serving size.  The "per serving size" of an item is often overlooked in the evaluation of food value.  For ice cream the 'per serving size' is ½ cup!!! For something to qualify as low carb just change the serving size! Indeed, this is what is going on with food products.  The manufacturers are simply reducing the portion size or serving size.  As such, they claim, it is now low carb.

The mind can be a very scary place when it comes to accounting.  If we used a food abusively when it was high carb, then we will use it abusively when it is low carb.  In a way, I think it is better to stay away from foods you have chronically abused whether they are low carb or not.  One other note, sugar alcohol has a laxative effect.  If one is over using products containing sugar alcohol, stay close to home. This particular laxative effect can be very unpredictable.

# Why You Can't Have Your Cake & Eat It, Too

## A Word About Seasonings

Be careful with any product that says it is sugar-free.  It will still contain carbohydrates.  Reading the label will be crucial in evaluating any product.  Many of the new sweeteners cook without losing sweetness.  Look for the syrups and sweeteners that are made with sucralose.  Here is a list of some suggested condiments:

Horseradish
Mustard
Soy sauce Lite
Salsa
Tabasco
Worcestershire
Butter Spray
Pam
Lemon juice
Limejuice
Vinegars, flavored
Dill pickles, relish
Olive Oil
Butter
Mayonnaise, real
Sour Cream
Guacamole
Real Ranch Dressing
Real Bleu Cheese Dressing

Foods containing sugar, honey, dextrose, sucrose, syrups, molasses, mannitol, maltitol, sugar alcohol, and sorbitol, will be prohibited due to their blood sugar elevating effect. Ketchups, barbeque sauce and spaghetti sauce will be loaded with sugar. Look for the new lo-carb products. Read the labels. Caution is advised.

## Appendix 6

### Evaluating Products

When looking for protein drinks, look at the label. You may live in an area that has different products than are available in a metropolitan area. Evaluate your protein drink based on the amount of protein it contains as well as the type. Most of the time, the protein drink will be made from whey protein, a very dense high grade of protein at 10 grams of protein per ounce. However, soy protein can be found in protein drinks. Some protein drinks contain both types of protein. The key in choosing a protein drink is its carbohydrate content. Some protein drinks contain a large amount of sugar from lactose or from syrups. These products will not be helpful in weight management. Ensure, Boost, or Slimfast are all examples of nutritional products that contain large amounts of sucrose. The marketing perception is directed to weight management through portion control. High glucose-containing products of any type are contrary to weight reduction strategies due to the stimulation of pancreatic insulin.

As you look at the label of these products, choose a high protein, low carbohydrate product. Remember to include the non-impact carbohydrates and count the fiber in the total carbohydrate counts. Non-impact carbohydrates and fiber do elevate blood sugar. Glycerol also elevates blood sugar and has a caloric value. These items will change as you look at the different products out in the market place. The food industry is scrambling to market its products in the low carb era, and they are introducing new products at a high rate of speed. In the period since 1999 there have been 450 new low carb products introduced, making regulation and testing very difficult. The low carb statement on a product does not give us confidence that a product will be truly low carb.

In human-based studies it has been demonstrated that sugar alcohol and fiber raise blood sugar. So the claim that sugar alcohol and fiber have a minimal effect on blood sugar is untrue. In my practice patients who check their blood sugars tell me that the so-called "zero carb" bars gave them elevations in their blood sugars. This is true for the "net carb" as well as the "zero carb" products.

Sweeteners will also vary in most protein drinks. Today Splenda is used more than aspartame in these products. Saccharin is not widely used in protein drinks or protein bars. Stevia and Splenda are the sweeteners used most often in high-protein low-carbohydrate products. These items tolerate heat and provide the sweetness we crave.

The sweetener Splenda is made from the sucrose molecule. It has been bombarded with chlorine gas and reduced in size 800 times. The smaller-size molecule means the sweetness factor is intensified with a smaller amount of product. This keeps the carbohydrate count down.

Stevia is made from yucca leaves. It is very sweet and powdery. In this form it acts just like sugar when used in cooking or sweetening food. Remember, Stevia is very sweet in small amounts. Stevia is also found in stores in a liquid form, handy for use in hot drinks or iced tea.

# Why You Can't Have Your Cake & Eat It, Too

Look for a protein drink containing at least 20 grams of protein.  Some protein drinks have 35 grams of protein or even 50 grams of protein.  The carbohydrate content should not be greater than 5 grams per container.  The selection you make should reflect these values.  Given the variables for individual preferences, it might be advantageous to try a couple of different protein drinks to find one you like.  Sweetness and texture factors can be enhanced with added protein powders or the DaVinci sugar free syrups.  Adding these items makes protein drinks more palatable.  For the vanilla protein drinks, adding instant coffee will turn it into an iced mocha frappachino.

The Internet has sites that provide protein drinks.  These sites will offer some significant savings on the purchase of larger quantities of products.  In the event you decide to purchase something from these sites, be sure you have taste-tested it first.  There are lots more high protein low carb low fat drinks out in the market place.  Be sure to read the label carefully and taste the product before you buy it in large quantities.

Sugar alcohols, contrary to what the food industry suggests, raises blood sugar.  This is easily demonstrated in individuals who are monitoring their blood sugars.  Sugar alcohols are also known as non-impact carbohydrates.  They do count in the overall carbohydrate values of the foods commonly known as "low-carb".  Be cautious with this type of food.  Count it as sugar related calories.

# Why You Can't Have Your Cake & Eat It, Too

## Ready or not

At this point you have enough information to get started. You will have to go to the grocery, health food store, and Trader Joe's (or another likeminded grocer). Gathering your supplies will be very important. Gauging how much is enough, what works, and what tastes good to you are going to be much more personal work. Getting feedback from your taste buds will help you figure out what you like and dislike. Soon you will be putting your plan into practice. At first it is fun, and then the old resistances will kick in. Over-analysis, second-guesses, postponing, and good old-fashioned worry will put you off the trail. Get started, ready or not.

## Appendix 7

**More Recipes**

**Richard Simmons Salad Dressing**

7 cups Fresh Salad Greens
! /2 cup chopped onion, celery, peppers, and mushrooms
Olive oil cooking spray
Vinegar of your Choice

Seasonings: oregano, parsley, pepper, salt, and artificial sweetener (ginger, mustard, are also good)

Spray the greens with the olive oil spray. Toss the seasonings and the sweetener into the salad. Pour your vinegar over the salad as desired.

One serving (3 ½ cups of salad) equals 5 Gms CHO. No fat.

Richard Simmons used to appear on TV doing his kookier exercise routines, along with a cooking segment. One day he offered this tip for making salad dressing. It really comes in handy at home. The olive oil spray makes the seasonings stick to the lettuces.

# Why You Can't Have Your Cake & Eat It, Too

## Strategic Hamburgers with Portobello Mushroom "Buns"

1 lb.  Super-lean ground beef, turkey, or chicken, formed into patties, seasoned as desired.  (3 or 4 patties. )

6 washed Portobello mushrooms sprayed with Olive oil and seasoned with garlic.

Grill the burger patties until desired doneness, grilling the mushrooms alongside the burgers.   Low fat cheese may be melted on the burgers to increase the protein.

Contains 32 Gms Protein,  8 Gms carbohydrate, 8 Gms fat.

 With added cheese go figure!

Optional idea: scrambled or poached eggs on the grilled mushrooms are another low carb way to enjoy eggs. Don't forget the salsa!!!

2 eggs=11gms Protein
Equivalent Egg Beaters = 10 Gms protein

## Oriental Stir Fry

1 pound Chicken tenders, washed and cleaned
1 bunch Green onions, Cleaned and chopped
1 pound cleaned fresh mushrooms
1 Bok choi cleaned and chopped into bite-size pieces
Ginger Paste
Minced Garlic
Oil for cooking

Sauce: ¾ cup cooking sherry, ¼ cup lite soy sauce, 2 Tbls cornstarch combined in a bowl with whisk.

Spray wok with non-stick cooking spray and begin heating. When hot, spread fresh ginger paste and the minced garlic on the sides on the pan.   Toss in the green onion first, then the mushrooms and the Bok choi.   Cook the veggies to desired doneness.  Fresh broccoli heads are also great with this dish. Remove veggies from the wok, and quickly add the chicken tenders, cooking them with added fresh ginger and garlic. When the tenders are cooked, move them to the edges of the wok.  Pour the sauce mix into the center of the hot wok.   It will thicken.   Return the veggies to the center of the wok into the bubbling sauce.  Fold in the chicken, and serve hot over steamed bean sprouts.  Note: other meats such as pork or beef may be used.  Serves four.

Contains per serving: Protein 32 Gms
                          Fat      4 Gms
                       CHO    5 Gms

## Strategically Placed Pumpkin Pie

2 packages of Mori Nu Lite Ex Firm Tofu (for a lighter texture the firm may be used)
2 cups of canned pumpkin
1-cup  sugar free maple-butter syrup or 2 cups Splenda
2 eggs
1 tsp vanilla
1 Tbsp Pumpkin pie spice or the next four ingredients
1 1/2 tsp cinnamon
2/3 tsp ground ginger
¼ tsp nutmeg
1/8 tsp ground cloves

Drain the tofu and blend in the food processor until smooth. Add remaining ingredients and blend well.  Spray a glass pie dish with cooking spray.  Pour the ingredients into the dish. Bake in a 350 F oven for one hour, at least.  Filling will be soft but it will firm up as it cools.  Chill and serve. Makes two pies. Serves 8.
One slice from 1/8 of the pie:
Protein 5 Gms
CHO     5 Gms
Fat     10 Gms

Phyllo dough may be used as crust, but the carbohydrate value will increase.  To use phyllo, cut the sheets in half, spray with cooking spray between layers, using up to four layers.  Made this way, the carbohydrate value is very low. Pour pie mix into the "crust" and bake.

# Why You Can't Have Your Cake & Eat It, Too

## Another Apple a Day, Strategically Speaking

One small apple, washed and cored
One-cup water
One tbsp vanilla
One cinnamon stick

2/3-cup low fat cottage cheese
One or two tablespoon of sugar free maple-butter syrup
Dash of cinnamon

Heat oven to 350 degrees.  Poke holes in the apple skin with a fork. Spray an ovenproof dish with non-stick vegetable spray and place the apple in it, with the cinnamon stick in the center. Combine water and vanilla and pour over the apple . Bake for 40-50 min. Remove from dish and set aside to cool, briefly.

In a bowl, combine the cottage cheese, and maple syrup. With the apple steaming hot, or cool, poor the cottage cheese atop, and sprinkle with cinnamon.  With the apple hot, the cheese will melt. Enjoy as a dessert, or breakfast.

Protein = 20 Gms
Carbohydrate =12 Gms

# Why You Can't Have Your Cake & Eat It, Too

## Recipes with Tofu

1 cake Mori Nu Tofu Lite (firm or extra firm)
2-3 tsp Crystal Lite granules,
Food processor needed.

Combine the ingredients in food processor with a blade until smooth and creamy.  This makes a wonderful breakfast, dessert, or anytime snack.

 Protein 20 Gms
CHO 8 Gms
Fat 4 Gms.

Tofu Variations:

Blend 1 cake of Mori Nu Tofu and 1 tsp sugar-free Jell-O granules in the food processor. Mix till creamy, eat and enjoy.

OR use 1 tbsp sugar-free instant pudding powder with 1 cake of Mori Nu Tofu in the food processor.    Mix until creamy. Note: the vanilla pudding mix with one-tablespoon instant coffee makes a yummy latte desert.

Smoothies:

2 scoops Protein Powder
1 can diet soda (root beer, strawberry, orange, or chocolate)
Ice.

 Combine in blender.  Enjoy!

# Why You Can't Have Your Cake & Eat It, Too

## Egg Drop Soup

2 cups Fat Free Chicken bouillon
3 eggs beaten
Green onion, mushroom, spinach
¼ tsp hot mustard

Heat soup until steaming, stir in eggs.  Add vegetables.  Stir in mustard.

## Savory Chicken Soup

4 Skinless boneless chicken breasts 4
1-quart fat-free chicken broth
1 each carrot, green onion, celery stick, leek, as bouquet
½ cup cooking sherry
Put all the above into a pot and cook until tender.  Strain the bouillon after the cooking is done and remove the bouquet. Add diced vegetables like green onion, peppers, and spinach. Steam until warm.  This is like a hot salad.  The chicken is good left over.

## Salmon Dip

1-Pound Smoked Salmon or canned
1-cup f low-fat cream cheese
½ cup chopped green onion
2 tbsp horseradish, ground
1 tsp liquid smoke

Combine above in food processor. Chill.
Assemble cucumber, celery, and green pepper crudités and use as dip.

# Why You Can't Have Your Cake & Eat It, Too

## Pancakes?

3 Eggs
1 tsp Vanilla
½ tsp baking soda
½ teas Cinnamon to taste
Stevia or Splenda to sweeten
½ cup cottage cheese
Sugar-Free Pancake syrup
Pam

Directions: Spray a large glass bowl with Pam.  Mix the first four ingredients in the bowl with a hand mixer.  Cover the mixture with a paper towel and microwave on high for 3 minutes or until cooked through.  When done, put it on a plate, add the cottage cheese, and drizzle with the Pancake syrup.

## Spaghetti Squash

Cut in half and clean out the seeds.  Set in glass dish.  Put a little water and cinnamon in the squash.  Cover with wax paper.  Microwave on high for 5 minutes.  Check for tenderness.  Microwave on high until done, 3-5 minutes. Separate the strands with a fork.

Using spaghetti squash instead of pasta is a low carb way to have your pasta and eat it too.  Steam the squash as above omitting the cinnamon.  Toss the strands with olive oil, chopped garlic, and Parmesan cheese.  Use a ¼ cup of stewed tomatoes.  All that is needed is a few meatballs or chicken.

## Lasagna

4 12 oz. Packages of Mori Nu Tofu Firm
Or 2 pounds of Precious Ricotta
1 ½ cup Mozzarella cheese, grated
2 large fresh eggs
1 large zucchini or eggplant
Parsley, pepper, garlic, oregano
1 large can Contadina crushed tomatoes
One pound ground beef or poultry

Blend the tofu or ricotta with the eggs and the spices. Sauté the meat till crumbly. Add the tomato to the meat and keep warm. Slice the eggplant or zucchini into strips, peeling them if you prefer. These vegetable strips will act as the pasta. Layer a 9 x 13 in. oiled glass dish with meat sauce followed by the vegetable strips, ricotta, and cheese with the top layer being vegetable strip. Cover the entire top with meat sauce. Bake covered in a 375-degree oven at least one hour. While still hot sprinkle more grated cheese on top. Ladle sauce over all to serve. 1/6 of pan is equal to 30 grams of protein and 7 grams of carbohydrate. It is better the next day.

## Appendix 8:
## Techniques that Work

### Road Work

Taking your diet with you means the incorporation of a lifestyle change under all conditions. Whether you work at home, in an office, or on the road, creating an environment for the continuous application of your eating strategies is a permanent commitment. This mission must thrive all the time. This will mean inclusive planning for vacations, holidays, reunions, tax season, and (especially) your birthday. Special events such as baseball games, going to the movies, and going to the theater require the same devotion to your health commitment. Planned or spontaneous, the special events of life will be enhanced with your efforts to hold on to your plan. Insulin resistance does not take a holiday. It is doing push ups in the gym, just waiting/weighting for a comeback tour of your metabolism.

The typical weight gain for a 2-week cruise is 8 pounds. Remember this is an average number of pounds gained. In my experience I have seen weight gains of 22 pounds in one week, in one person who ventured off plan. This is not the only example of many insulin-resistant clients in my practice. Try to keep in your mind the irreversible nature of insulin resistance. Together we can achieve a degree of manageability over it. As the fat mass in the abdomen is reduced, many wonderful experiences that have been postponed will become available to you.

This is especially true in the trying times of life as well. It is not easy to maintain your healthy commitments during stressful times.   Take your difficult times as an opportunity to develop confidence in your ability to adapt to the circumstances as they come.  You can do it, I believe in you.

Planning for air travel is always a challenge. Standing in lines, going through security, and the uncertainty create added stress. Getting to the airport with time to spare is an advantage.  Take a liter of bottled water with you. Be sure to drink it while you are in the airport. Obtain a spare bottle before you board the aircraft.   These can be purchased chilled at the airport concessions.   While in flight you can obtain hot water from the service personnel for making herbal tea.  Bring your special flavor as a delightful change of taste. Remember high altitudes are very dehydrating.   This is especially true during airplane travel as well as during visits to high altitude communities.  Most of us have experienced the unpleasant "irregularity" that accompanies travel. This can be managed by maintaining your water intake.  .

Jerky is just about the best thing invented for having high quality protein food with you.    This tip is not just for travel. Keeping some turkey jerky on hand all the time will keep you on track when your options for healthful dieting get limited.  If you find a deli at the airport, have them make you a sandwich with double portions of meat.  Be sure to throw away the bread or bagel if it comes that way.  More and more, we are seeing food service that is amenable to us high-protein dieters.    Various hamburger establishments are willing to make protein burgers, which consist of one or two hamburger patties with cheese and dill pickle wrapped in iceberg lettuce. This option also works for fajitas or hot dogs.  It can happen!

# Why You Can't Have Your Cake & Eat It, Too

Avoid the lure of fat-free yogurt and frozen coffee beverages. A Grande iced mocha using non-fat milk will contain 33 grams of carbohydrates, and more if you add chocolate and sugar. Remember, if it says fat-free it is not fat, and for sure not protein. It is mainly sugar.

Going from home to work will require some alterations in the way you manage the pacing of your diet. The deli-style protein is just about the best thing going for the "grab and go" culture. There are some delicious deli style meats at your grocers. Repacking the meat slices into 4-ounce Baggies works the best. Many delicatessens will be happy to do this for you at the time you buy it. Cheese might be different, but adding a few slices to the bag will be good. Often salads can be purchased at the same time. The pre-sliced celery, peppers, and radishes will complement the meal you have created. Avoid those baby carrots. They weigh in at 2 carbs per carrot. It won't take long for them to add up.

Be careful with bread and starches for they can contain large volumes of carbohydrates. Today's bread suppliers are creating some interesting choices for "low carb" bread, bagel, and tortillas. Remember to look for the total number of carbs in the item, not the net grams of carbs.

Cans of protein drinks should be served cold. Keep your supply stocked. For added taste look for the DaVinci sugar-free syrups as a flavor enhancer. A teaspoon or two of instant coffee softened with a touch of water can be added to chocolate or vanilla protein drinks. Now this mocha latte java isn't going to crash the diet. Protein powders can be mixed into the protein drinks. This is called "spiking." A technique like this can boost your protein intake if you have fallen behind in your daily counts. Vanilla protein powders in diet orange soda or diet root beer whip into a really awesome smoothie. Try a protein drink in the car on the ride home after a long day. You might find you aren't as hungry when you get to your destination.

Cottage cheese is a most adaptable food. Serving it with cinnamon and sweetener makes a high-protein sweet snack. Served it with ranch dressing mix, it becomes a terrific dip for vegetables. Cottage cheese melts in a topping-type situation for baked apples or broiled tomatoes. Hard-boiled eggs are another example of a great fast food. They are great for packing along or for storing in the refrigerator. They just need to be made up ahead of time.

For special occasions plan to have something to celebrate, your continued state of health! Sugar-free Jell-O with whipped cream is a good idea. Strawberries or berries in general are good, alone or served with whipped cream or sour cream. There are some frozen deserts in the form of frozen bars, which claim to be fat-free. As usual, they contain carbohydrates and are sweetened with things like aspartame or sucralose. Look for items with the lowest carbohydrate value. Your local grocer may have an ample supply to choose from. There are sugar-free Popsicles containing 4 to 6 calories per single pop. There are sorbets available with some low carbohydrate values as well. The serving sizes are small. It is important to be aware what constitutes a serving size. As with the low carb bread, be sure to count the total carbs, not the net carbs, when considering the frozen confections.

# Why You Can't Have Your Cake & Eat It, Too

Advance planning is necessary when using these foods.  Look at your consumption of protein.  Remember your carbohydrate tolerances must consider the amount selected for your continued weight management.  Consider also the severity of symptoms when choosing carbohydrates.  Then, by using some evaluation techniques you will be able to make an informed choice.

Occasionally someone will ask if it is okay to use sugar-free pie on this type of diet.  The short answer is no.  The long answer is about the number of carbohydrate calories per slice. Fruit, flour, juice, and fat all contain a large amount of calories. The caloric value in sugar-free pie is related to the carbohydrates and fat in the total recipe.  Divide the number of servings per pie, and you can just about figure out the caloric and carbohydrate expense per slice.  It is possible to reduce the total calories per slice with the sugar-free technique, but  be mindful of the grams of carbohydrates.

Be very careful with consuming these things late in the evening.  These types of foods may cause overnight high blood sugar.  When the blood sugar is high during the night, fat oxidation is interrupted.  Sleep is a fat-burning activity and we must do what we can to promote it.  Keeping the blood sugar at lowered levels promotes fat oxidation.  Stored body fat is a constant energetic source of fuel.

An item containing 20 grams of carbohydrates can be viewed with other similar foods.  A one-ounce piece of bread is equal to one Hagen-Das chocolate sorbet stick.  This is a judgment you will have to make.  From my perspective it is not a good idea to have sorbet everyday.

# Why You Can't Have Your Cake & Eat It, Too

Remember, if you have abused ice cream in the past, your capacity to abuse it now is still there.  This axiom is true for the sugar-free items now available at the market.  We are trying to develop good skills in the rationing of all foods.  This type of skill development will be instrumental in the creation of a sense of well being, self-esteem, and connectedness.  Try to be willing to experiment with new foods, new preparation methods, and new menus.  This will add freshness to your diet.

## Counter-Top Grilling

This is one of the best inventions for grilling meats and vegetables in the home.  The many different brands of these counter top grillers come with a non-stick surface and a tray for catching the drippings.  Clean up is a breeze, provided you unplug it first and apply wet paper towels to the cooking surfaces.  After such soaking on the surfaces, the paper towels will wipe away the residue.

Using your favorite counter top griller you can quickly cook many different types of protein.  Swordfish, pork chops, and chicken do very well on the grill, as do Portobello mushrooms and eggplant.  Steaks are particularly good cooked in this way.  Crab cakes or hamburger patties are done in a flash.  When the weather is too hot or too cold for outside grilling you can still grill indoors with the counter-top griller.

If you have a glass-top stove, you will find this a good spot to set up your grill.  Then you can use the hood for ventilation.  This is a good surface in general for hot appliances when there may be cooking spatter.

There are many applications for cooking your favorite protein food on the portable counter-top grill.  A good suggestion is to cook more than one serving at a time.  Leftovers can be stored in the refrigerator for quick heat-and-eat meals the next day.  Cheeseburgers, salmon burgers, and chicken breast work great this way.

## Crispy Canadian Bacon

Remember the days we cooked bacon in the microwave?  It would get crispy.  We used it in many ways, not all of them healthful.  A good idea was passed along to me from one of my clients.  Canadian bacon, thinly cut ham, can be cooked in this way as well.  Cook it on high for one minute per slice.  This crispy ham can be crumbled on salads, or used in omelets.  It is quite salty, so If you have a problem with salt, you may want to find meats that are not heavily salted.

## Steaming Vegetables

Another handy technique for cooking veggies is to steam them or cook them using fat-free chicken broth or beef broth. The broth seasons the food and you won't need butter.

The flavors of cooking sprays are useful in the seasoning of your vegetables.  Spraying them with the butter flavor is a fat saver and a flavor booster.  The olive oil spray is especially nice on salads.

## Meals ready to Eat

Convenience foods like the 'MRE's" are available in the meat counters. Choices like pot-roast, roasted chicken, roast turkey, pork loin roast, and meatballs can be found there. These items are pre-cooked in nice gravy and happen to be quite good. They require heating for very short times. As with most of these foods, be careful if there are added breadcrumbs or rice. This will have a serious impact on blood sugar and weight loss.

# Why You Can't Have Your Cake & Eat It, Too

## Food Record Sample

Day                            Date

| Food/Drink Item | Am't | Fat | Carb | Prot | H2O |
|---|---|---|---|---|---|
|  |  |  |  |  |  |
|  |  |  |  |  |  |
|  |  |  |  |  |  |
|  |  |  |  |  |  |
|  |  |  |  |  |  |
|  |  |  |  |  |  |
|  |  |  |  |  |  |
|  |  |  |  |  |  |
|  |  |  |  |  |  |
|  |  |  |  |  |  |
|  |  |  |  |  |  |
|  |  |  |  |  |  |
|  |  |  |  |  |  |
|  |  |  |  |  |  |
| Daily Totals |  |  |  |  |  |

## Why You Can't Have Your Cake & Eat It, Too

Use this form to record your food intake.  To self-monitor your progress food records are most helpful.  Some Internet sites will have food records you could use, and food composition.  This will give you a reflection of your work.  Food records will help you as you work with a professional nutrition coach.  Together you will be able to calculate your nutritional values, and your water intake.  If corrections need to be made, or progress is stalled, the food record will give clear signs of what direction is necessary.

# Why You Can't Have Your Cake & Eat It, Too

## Thoughts

Food-borne illness has been the province of bacteria and viruses. Disease obtained from contaminated food or improper cleaning of food will contribute considerable distress. These symptoms will be entirely unpleasant. They arrive suddenly, have a noted ferocity, and dissipate with prompt attention. If appropriate preventative measures are taken, then these types of problems will not return.

In this time, food borne illness has become more expansive. We know that inappropriate eating can cause zillions of problems as varied as the stars in the sky. Given the individual nature of heredity and lifestyle, the effects of these inappropriate eating styles can be entirely unpleasant. They may arrive slowly, have an annoying quality, and with inattention grow into serious life threatening chronic disease.

Chronic disease is just one outcome to these food borne diseases. The expense of treatment is enormous and must be obtained from professionals. Expensive pharmaceuticals are often required as over the counter remedies will not be of help.

Yet, there is much I can do as individuals to prevent, and to avoid the harmful effects of a destructive eating style. This we must do if we are to outrun the consequences of our lifestyles.


Blessings and Joy,

Nadine Campbell, R.N.

# Why You Can't Have Your Cake & Eat It, Too



## Benediction

"We seek a renewed stirring of life for the earth
We plead that what we are capable of doing is not
Always what we ought to do.
We urge that all people now determine
That a wide untrammeled freedom shall remain
To testify that this generation has love for the next.
If we want to succeed in that, we might show, meanwhile
A little more love for this one, and each other."

Nancy Newhall

**To order books:**

Mail request to or call:

Nutritional Strategies
4659 S Lakeshore Dr #E
Tempe, AZ 85282
480 831 9105

Please include Check for $20, plus $6 for shipping and handling.